T0265387

The Biology of
Multiple Sclerosis

The Biology of Multiple Sclerosis

Gregory J. Atkins
Fellow Emeritus of the Department of Microbiology, Moyne Institute of Preventive Medicine,
Trinity College Dublin, Dublin, Ireland

Sandra Amor
Professor and Head of MS Research, Pathology Department, VU Medical Center, Amsterdam, The Netherlands

Jean M. Fletcher
Assistant Professor at the Schools of Medicine and Biochemistry and Immunology,
Trinity Biomedical Sciences Institute, Trinity College Dublin, Dublin, Ireland

Kingston H.G. Mills
Professor at the School of Biochemistry and Immunology, Trinity Biomedical Sciences Institute,
Trinity College Dublin, Dublin, Ireland

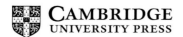

CAMBRIDGE
UNIVERSITY PRESS

CAMBRIDGE
UNIVERSITY PRESS

University Printing House, Cambridge CB2 8BS, United Kingdom

Cambridge University Press is part of the University of Cambridge.

It furthers the University's mission by disseminating knowledge in the pursuit of education, learning and research at the highest international levels of excellence.

www.cambridge.org
Information on this title: www.cambridge.org/9780521196802

First published 2012

A catalogue record for this publication is available from the British Library

Library of Congress Cataloguing in Publication data

The biology of multiple sclerosis / Gregory J. Atkins . . . [et al.].
   p. cm.
ISBN 978-0-521-19680-2 (Hardback)
1. Multiple sclerosis. I. Atkins, Gregory J.
RC377.B55 2012
616.8´34–dc23

                                         2012020427

ISBN 978-0-521-19680-2 Hardback

Contents

Contributors

David Baker
Blizard Institue, Barts and the London
School of Medicine and Dentistry,
Queen Mary University of London,
London, UK

Brian Sheahan
Professor Emeritus, Veterinary Sciences
Centre, UCD School of Agriculture, Food
Science and Veterinary Medicine,
University College Dublin, Belfield,
Dublin, Ireland

Paul van der Valk
Pathology Department,
VU Medical Center, Amsterdam,
The Netherlands

Preface

Multiple sclerosis (MS) is the most common debilitating neurological disease in relatively young people (less than 40 years old) in developed countries; in these countries it has a prevalence of around 1 in 800. It is a disease characterised by focal lymphocytic infiltration of the brain and spinal cord leading to damage to myelin, and eventually also to axons. The most common clinical course of the disease is relapsing and remitting, leading to a progressive course, but in about 10% of patients the disease is initially progressive (primary progressive MS). In both forms of the disease, there is usually progressive neurological disability, but patients may survive for many years.

Investigation of the cause and characteristics of MS has been the subject of intensive research effort; although at least one partially successful treatment has been developed, the cause of MS is still unknown. A large body of evidence suggests that autoimmunity is involved. Studies of the epidemiology and genetics of MS suggest an interaction between an environmental factor and genetic susceptibility.

The clinical aspects of MS have been well covered in other publications. Our aim here is to review the scientific literature that has been published on the biology of MS, and to provide a scientific overview.

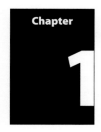

Chapter

1

Introduction: the biological basis

Gregory J. Atkins

History of discovery

Throughout the course of history, people have been ill with diseases affecting their mobility. This could take the form of increasing paralysis over time. For many, this was associated with other symptoms, such as numbness, dizziness, and blurred vision. In the eighteenth century, physicians began to classify such cases into broad groups. The term paraplegia was used for people who had progressive paralysis. A major advance was made in 1868 by the physician Jean-Martin Charcot and his colleague Edmé Vulpian. They studied the tremors of younger patients and differentiated a condition from that described by James Parkinson in 1817. At autopsy such patients were found to have grey patches (plaques) scattered throughout the spinal cord and brain. Charcot gave a series of lectures on the features of this disease, which he termed *sclérose en plaque disseminée* and which we now know as multiple sclerosis (MS). Since then, a large amount of research has been carried out on this disease, and much progress has been made in understanding its pathogenesis. However, the primary cause of the disease still remains elusive (1).

Characteristics of the disease

MS is an inflammatory disease of the human central nervous system (CNS) leading to damage to myelin and axons; this damage occurs in localised plaques. Early in the disease demyelination of myelinated axons is followed by remyelination leading to transient recovery, but later extensive and chronic neurodegeneration occurs, including axonal loss, leading to irreversible disability.

MS occurs in three forms: relapsing and remitting (about 90% of cases), primary progressive (about 10% of cases), and secondary progressive (derived from relapsing–remitting). Relapsing and remitting MS is characterised by clinical episodes, which may be of progressive severity, interspersed by periods of stability. In primary progressive MS the course of the disease is continuous from the onset. Secondary progressive MS develops later in the course of the relapsing–remitting disease, usually 6–10 years after onset.

The age of onset of MS is usually between 20 and 40 years, making it the most common cause of neurological disability in young adults in areas of high prevalence, although childhood MS also occurs. Except for a minority with aggressive MS, life expectancy for MS patients is near normal. Although the majority of MS patients experience progressive disability, a minority has benign MS in which progression of the disease has halted.

The Biology of Multiple Sclerosis, ed Gregory J. Atkins, Sandra Amor, Jean M. Fletcher and Kingston H.G. Mills. Published by Cambridge University Press. © Gregory J. Atkins, Sandra Amor, Jean M. Fletcher and Kingston H.G. Mills 2012.

The prevalence of MS is highest among white populations in temperate regions, and in Europe and North America it is 1/800. Multiple sclerosis is thus a common disease in developed countries. However, it is clear from epidemiological studies that it shows regional variation in prevalence, that clusters have occurred, and that there is a genetic basis to MS. Study of these phenomena has provided circumstantial evidence concerning the etiology of MS, although the evidence from any one aspect may be tenuous and often contradictory (see reference (2) for a general review of MS). It is therefore necessary to take an overview of the factors involved in the etiology of MS and to formulate a general hypothesis, before specific etiological agents are considered.

Diagnosis
Clinical signs
Most patients present with an acute episode affecting one (or occasionally several) site (Table 1.1); the symptoms increase in number and severity with time.

Electrophoresis of the cerebral spinal fluid (CSF) shows the presence of oligoclonal bands of immunoglobulin in MS patients, although this is only diagnostic in conjunction with other criteria such as those shown in Table 1.1 and magnetic resonance imaging (MRI). However, there are no other reliable biomarkers for the progression of disease in MS (3).

Magnetic resonance imaging
In 1981 an advance was made in the diagnosis of MS by the first description of MS lesions detected by MRI (Figure 1.1) (4). It was later confirmed that MRI corresponds to lesions in the brain from studies of autopsy tissue (5). During the 1990s, drug studies in MS incorporated MRI assessment, providing information about the underlying disease (1). However, it was clear that the changes that resemble MS lesions could occur in other conditions, and also in apparently healthy people, so MRI is not a sole diagnostic criterion but is correlated with other clinical signs occurring in the patient. Repeated MRIs on the same patient showed that the disease has continuous activity, even when the patient is not experiencing new symptoms, and computer models were developed to measure disease burden based on the number and volume of lesions (6).

In 1986 it was shown that the enhancing agent gadolinium-DPTA caused some lesions to enhance whereas others did not. The enhancement identified breakdown of the blood–brain barrier, indicating areas of inflammation (7). Thus gadolinium enhancement has become a useful technique to demonstrate new and active MS lesions, effectively monitoring disease activity (8).

Autopsy
The diagnostic tests mentioned above are not specific, but are used in conjunction with clinical findings to reach a diagnosis. However, the final and unequivocal diagnosis of MS is by autopsy. The characteristic changes noted in the CNS at autopsy are scattered lesions in the white matter (plaques), with the features of inflammation (Figure 1.2), demyelination, some axonal damage, and gliosis.

Evidence for an environmental factor
Some of the earliest studies on the prevalence and epidemiology of MS are the immigration studies carried out by Dean and colleagues (9–12). Although the numbers of patients used were small, immigration to the UK from the Indian subcontinent and the Caribbean, and

Table 1.1 Symptoms of MS

Site affected	Symptoms
Cerebrum	Cognitive impairment Hemisensory and motor Affective (mainly depression) Epilepsy (rare) Focal cortical deficits (rare)
Optic nerve	Unilateral painful loss of vision
Cerebellum	Tremor Clumsiness and poor balance
Brainstem	Diplopia, oscillopsia Vertigo Impaired swallowing Impaired speech and emotional lability Paroxysmal symptoms
Spinal cord	Weakness Stiffness and painful spasms Bladder dysfunction Erectile impotence Constipation
Other	Pain Fatigue Temperature sensitivity and exercise intolerance

Derived in part from (2).

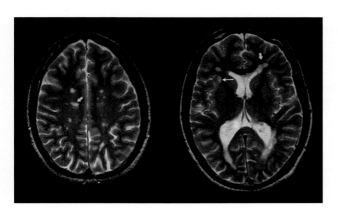

Figure 1.1. Two representative T2-weighted MR images of an MS patient. Thick arrows indicate typical periventricular (round or ovoid) white matter lesions; thin arrow in the right panel indicates a juxtacortical lesion in the insula region.

from other countries to South Africa, was studied (Figure 1.3A). On the basis of this data, it was postulated that immigration before the age of puberty results in a prevalence of MS reflecting the region of origin, whereas immigration after the age of puberty results in a prevalence in keeping with the destination region. This has been interpreted as indicating that an environmental factor exerts its effect at or around the age of puberty.

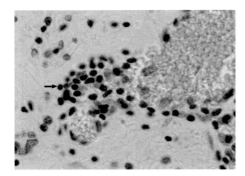

Figure 1.2. This MS autopsy section shows a vessel filled with red blood cells and surrounded by lymphocytes (arrow). Haematoxylin and eosin × 60. (Courtesy Dr. F. Brett, Beaumont Hospital, Dublin.)

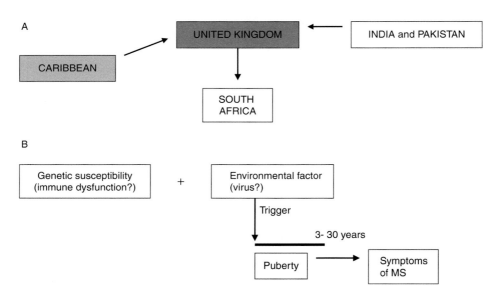

Figure 1.3. Diagrammatic representation of the immigration studies carried out by Dean and others and the hypothesis derived from these and other studies. (A) Some regions involved in the immigration studies; prevalence of MS is proportional to the degree of shading. (B) Schematic diagram showing how the interaction between an environmental factor and genetic susceptibility could result in MS.

This hypothesis has been substantiated by a study of Caribbean immigrants moving to France and their return migration (13,14), but is not consistent with a study of UK and Irish immigrants moving to Australia (15).

Consistent with the idea of an environmental factor is the occurrence of 'clusters' of MS. Very generally, the prevalence of MS varies by latitude, being most common further away from the equator (about 1 in 800 in Northern Europe and Australia). Clusters of MS have been described in Iceland, Key West (Florida), and the Faroe Islands and smaller divergences in prevalence have been found in several other areas. In the Faroe Islands, the increase in incidence of MS occurred following the occupation of the islands for 5 years by British troops during the Second World War. Multiple sclerosis on the Faroe Islands occurred in four successive epidemics after 1943. It has been postulated

Table 1.2 Viruses that have been implicated in the etiology of multiple sclerosis

Virus	Family	Nucleic acid
Measles	Paramyxovirus	RNA(−ve)
Rubella	Togavirus	RNA(+ve)
Epstein–Barr	Herpesvirus	DNA
Varicella-zoster	Herpesvirus	DNA
Herpes 6	Herpesvirus	DNA
Endogenous retrovirus	Retrovirus	RNA/DNA*

*RNA replicated via DNA integrated into the genome, or present as a DNA copy (provirus) integrated into the genome and replicated with the cellular DNA.

that this occurred through the spread of an unknown infectious agent which is asymptomatic and which triggered MS in only a minority of infections. Clearly this could have been a virus introduced by the British troops, but this has not been unequivocally established (16).

Nature of the environmental factor

Most studies have concentrated on identifying a virus infection as the trigger for MS. Some studies have suggested other environmental factors in the etiology of MS. These include smoking, diet, and bacteria (17–20). There is also a possible influence of sunlight and vitamin D.

Viruses

Several viruses have been implicated, including measles virus, rubella virus, Epstein-Barr virus, varicella-zoster virus, human herpesvirus type 6, and human retrovirus (Table 1.2).

Unspecified infections (mainly respiratory tract infections), occurring before relapses of MS, have also been implicated (17). The evidence for the involvement of specific viruses will be reviewed in Chapter 6.

Vitamin D

The hypothesis that vitamin D deficiency is a risk factor for MS is based on the immuno-modulatory effects of vitamin D (21). The hypothesis of an increased risk among individuals with low vitamin D concentrations derives from epidemiological evidence similar to that described above, i.e. that the risk for both MS and vitamin D deficiency may be related to sunlight exposure (see reference 22 for a general review).

Vitamin D is available from two sources: skin exposure to ultraviolet B (UVB) radiation in sunlight and diet (Figure 1.4). Compared to UVB exposure, diet (e.g. fatty fish) is a poor source of vitamin D. Vitamin D is biologically inactive and is converted in the liver to 25-hydroxyvitamin D. This then undergoes a second hydroxylation in the kidney or other tissues to give the active form, 1,25-dihydroxyvitamin D. This binds and activates the vitamin D receptor (VDR), a transcription factor that regulates the expression of as many as 500 genes (23). These include the regulation of calcium physiology, effects on

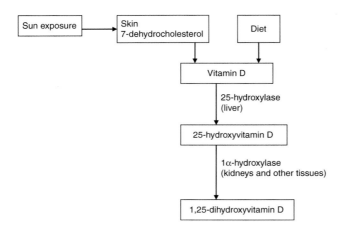

Figure 1.4. Origins and metabolism of vitamin D. Derived in part from (21).

brain development and function, regulation of blood pressure and insulin secretion, and particularly in this context, effects on the differentiation of immune cells and modulation of immune responses (24).

The reasons that vitamin D deficiency may be a risk factor for MS are based on: (1) the fact that MS frequency generally increases with increasing latitude, which is inversely correlated with duration and intensity of UVB from sunlight and vitamin D concentrations; (2) the fact that the prevalence of MS is lower than expected at high latitudes in populations with high consumption of fatty fish, which is high in vitamin D (25); and (3) the data on MS risk associated with migration (described above).

If vitamin D has an effect on MS risk, MS incidence would be expected to decrease with increasing serum 25-hydroxyvitamin D concentrations. It is known that 25-hydroxyvitamin D concentrations decline after MS onset (26). One longitudinal study on 25-hydroxyvitamin D concentrations before the onset of MS has been conducted (27). This sampled a cohort from 7 million individuals from the US military who had at least two serum samples stored. Individuals with more than 99.2 nmol/l 25-hydroxyvitamin D (top quintile) had a 62% lower odds of developing MS than those in the bottom quintile (less than 63.3 nmol/l). Thus it was concluded that the serum concentration of 25-hydroxyvitamin D in healthy white adults is a predictor of their risk of developing MS. This association could be due either to a true protective effect of vitamin D or confounded by a factor affecting both 25-hydroxyvitamin D concentration and MS risk, such as UVB exposure, which could have immunosuppressive effects.

In another study, using 200 000 women, vitamin D intake was measured every 4 years by a comprehensive food frequency questionnaire (28). The validity of the estimated vitamin D intake was assessed in a subgroup of 300. The incidence of MS during the 30-year follow-up decreased with increasing vitamin D intake (p=0.03) and was 33% lower among women in the highest quintile compared to those in the lowest. Thus it can be concluded that vitamin D intake is a predictor of MS risk.

A further study has analysed 132 patients with MS, 58 with relapsing–remitting MS (RRMS) during remission, 34 RRMS patients during relapse, and 40 primary progressive MS cases (PPMS). Sixty healthy individuals matched with respect to place of residence, race/ethnicity, age, and gender were used as controls. Levels of 25-hydroxyvitamin D and

1,25-dihydroxyvitamin D were lower in RRMS patients than in controls. Also, levels in patients suffering relapses were lower than those during remissions. PPMS patients showed similar values to controls. Proliferation of both freshly isolated CD4+ T cells and MBP-specific T cells was inhibited by 1,25-dihydroxyvitamin D. T cells were able to metabolise 25-hydroxyvitamin D into biologically active 1,25-dihydroxyvitamin D, since T cells express 1α-hydroxylase constitutively (29).

A protective effect of vitamin D is in agreement with most data on the geographical distribution of MS, including the latitude gradient, although the data is not yet unequivocal. A Canadian study has shown no apparent association between vitamin D metabolic pathway genes and MS susceptibility (30). However, one study has identified weak evidence of an association between a common variation within the vitamin D receptor gene and MS (31).

It has been suggested that population-wide diet supplementation programmes might be a prevention strategy for MS (32). However, diet supplementation with vitamin D to prevent not only MS but other diseases has been questioned. A panel put together by the Institute of Medicine has issued a report that challenged this view. They asserted that blood levels of vitamin D need not be as high as had been advocated, and high doses of the vitamin could actually cause harm (33).

Evidence for a genetic factor

MS is more common in White people than in other racial groups, and is also more common in women than men. It has a higher familial risk in first- or second-degree relatives than unrelated individuals (2,34), and monozygotic twins have a higher concordance rate than dizygotic twins (2,35). These facts taken together indicate a genetic predisposition to MS.

Further evidence for a genetic basis for MS susceptibility has been obtained by studying the association between MS and alleles of the multiple histocompatibility complex. Initially, a relationship was established between MS and genotypes HLA-DRB1, HLA-DRB5, HLA-DQA1, and HLA-DQB2 (2,36). This relationship holds for most Europeans except some Mediterranean groups. More recently, it has been shown that a complex epistatic interaction between HLA-DRB1, HLA-DQA1, and HLA-DQB1 determines susceptibility to MS (37). A genomewide study of risk alleles for MS using microarray technology has identified alleles of the interleukin-2 receptor alpha gene, interleukin-7 receptor alpha gene, and multiple alleles in the HLA locus as heritable risk factors (38). In a collaborative study involving 9772 cases of European descent collected by 23 research groups working in 15 different countries, almost all of the previously suggested associations were replicated and at least a further 29 susceptibility loci identified (39). Within the MHC the identity of the HLA-DRB1 risk alleles was refined. Immunologically relevant genes were significantly over-represented among those mapping close to the identified loci, and T helper cell differentiation was particularly implicated in the pathogenesis of MS. These studies indicate that susceptibility to MS is probably polygenic and the result of complex interactions between alleles.

Disease mechanisms

The primary disease lesions in MS are sclerotic plaques that occur in the brain and spinal cord. These are areas of inflammation, demyelination, and neuronal degeneration that probably result from increased migration of autoreactive lymphocytes across the blood–brain barrier (2). These disease processes result in loss of axonal conduction. The immune specificity of the autoreactive lymphocytes has not yet been determined, although there have been many proposals. The main problem is that autoreactive lymphocytes are also present in normal individuals, but it has been shown that regulatory lymphocytes from MS patients fail to suppress effector cells (40).

Detailed studies of the pathology of MS lesions from a large number of patients indicate that a number of different mechanisms of demyelination may operate (41,42). It is possible therefore that MS may be a disease with a number of different etiologies, all of which have a common pathological end point.

Conclusion

A generally accepted mechanism for the etiology of MS is that the disease results from interaction between an environmental factor and genetic susceptibility (Figure 1.3B), although the environmental factor is still unknown and the genetics is complex. It is not known how the genetic determinants of the disease result in the disease phenotype.

References

1. Murray, T.J. (2005). *Multiple Sclerosis: The History of a Disease*. Demos Medical Publishing, New York.

2. Compston, A. and Coles, A. (2008). Multiple sclerosis. *Lancet* **372**, 1502–1517.

3. Grabera, J.J. and Dhib-Jalbut, S. (2011). Biomarkers of disease activity in multiple sclerosis. *J. Neurol. Sci.* **305**, 1–10.

4. Young, I.R., Hall, A.S., Pallis, C.A., *et al.* (1981). Nuclear magnetic resonance imaging of the brain in multiple sclerosis. *Lancet* **318**, 1063–1066.

5. Ormerod, I.E., Miller, D.H., McDonald, W.I., *et al.* (1987). The role of NMR imaging in the assessment of multiple sclerosis and isolated neurological lesions: a quantitative study. *Brain* **110**, 1579–1616.

6. Inglese, M., Grossman, R.I., and Filippi, M. (2005). Magnetic resonance imaging monitoring of multiple sclerosis lesion evolution. *J. Neuroimaging* **15**, 22S–29S.

7. Grossman, R.I., Gonzalez-Scarano, F., Atlas, S.W., Galetta, S., and Silberberg, D.H. (1986). Multiple sclerosis: gadolinium enhancement in MR imaging. *Radiology* **161**, 721–725.

8. Katz, D., Taubenberger, J.K., Cannella, B., *et al.* (1993). Correlation between magnetic resonance imaging findings and lesion development in chronic, active multiple sclerosis. *Ann. Neurol.* **34**, 661–669.

9. Dean, G. and Elian, M. (1997). Age at immigration to England of Asian and Caribbean immigrants and the risk of developing multiple sclerosis. *J. Neurol. Neurosurg. Psychiatry* **63**, 565–568.

10. Elian, M. and Dean, G. (1993). Motor neuron disease and multiple sclerosis among immigrants to England from the Indian subcontinent, the Caribbean, and east and west Africa. *J. Neurol. Neurosurg. Psychiatry* **56**, 454–457.

11. Elian, M., Nightingale, S., and Dean, G. (1990). Multiple sclerosis among United Kingdom-born children of immigrants from the Indian subcontinent, Africa and the West Indies. *J. Neurol. Neurosurg. Psychiatry* **53**, 906–911.

12. Dean G. and Kurtzke, J.F. (1971). On the risk of multiple sclerosis according to age at immigration to South Africa. *Br. Med. J.* **3**, 725–729.

13. Cabre, P. (2007). Migration and multiple sclerosis: the French West Indies experience. *J. Neurol. Sci.* **262**, 117–121.

14. Cabre, P., Signate, A., Olindo, S., *et al.* (2005). Role of return migration in the emergence of multiple sclerosis in the French West Indies. *Brain* **128**, 2899–2910.

15. Hammond, S.R., English, D.R., and McLeod, J.G. (2000). The age-range of risk of developing multiple sclerosis: evidence from a migrant population in Australia. *Brain* **123**, 968–974.

16. Kurtzke, J.F. (2000). Multiple sclerosis in time and space: geographic clues to cause. *J. Neurovirol.* **Suppl 2**:S134–140.

17. Buljevac, D., Flack, H.Z., Hop W.C.J., *et al.* (2002). Prospective study on the relationship between infections and multiple sclerosis exacerbations. *Brain* **125**, 952–960.

18. Hernan, M.A., Jick, S.S., Longroscino, G., *et al.* (2005). Cigarette smoking and the progression of multiple sclerosis. *Brain* **128**, 1461–1465.

19. Marrie, R.A. (2004). Environmental risk factors in multiple sclerosis. *Lancet Neurol.* **3**, 709–718.

20. Stratton, C.W. and Wheldon, D.B. (2006). Multiple sclerosis: an infectious syndrome involving *Chlamydophila pneumoniae*. *Trends Microbiol.* **14**, 474–479.

21. Hayes, C.E., Cantorna, M.T., and Deluca, H.F. (1997). Vitamin D and multiple sclerosis. *Proc. Soc. Exp. Biol. Med.* **216**, 21–27.

22. Ascherio, A., Munger, K., and Simon, K.C. (2010). Vitamin D and multiple sclerosis. *Lancet Neurol.* **9**, 599–612.

23. Norman, A.W. (2006). Vitamin D receptor (VDR): new assignments for an already busy receptor. *Endocrinology* **147**, 5542–5548.

24. Deluca, H.F. and Cantorna, M.T. (2001). Vitamin D: its role and uses in immunology. *FASEB J.* **15**, 2579–2585.

25. Swank, R.L, Lerstad, O., Strom, A., and Backer, J. (1952). Multiple sclerosis in rural Norway: its geographic and occupational incidence in relation to nutrition. *N. Engl. J. Med.* **246**, 721–728.

26. Correale, J., Ysrraelit, M.C., and Gaitan, M.I. (2009). Immunomodulatory effects of vitamin D in multiple sclerosis. *Brain* **132**, 1146–1160.

27. Munger, K.L., Levin, L.I., Hollis, B.W., Howard, N.S., and Ascherio, A. (2006). Serum 25-hydroxyvitamin D levels and risk of multiple sclerosis. *JAMA* **296**, 2832–2838.

28. Feskanich, D., Willett, W.C., and Colditz, G.A. (2003). Calcium, vitamin D, milk consumption, and hip fractures: a prospective study among postmenopausal women. *Am. J. Clin. Nutr.* **77**, 504–511.

29. Correale, J., Ysrraellt, M.C., and Galtan, M.I. (2011). Vitamin D-mediated immune regulation in multiple sclerosis. *J. Neurol. Sci.* **311**, 23–31.

30. Orton, S., Sreeram, V.R., Para, A.E., *et al.* (2011). Vitamin D metabolic pathway genes and risk of multiple sclerosis in Canadians. *J. Neurol. Sci.* **305**, 116–120.

31. Cox, M.B., Ban, M., Bowden, N.A., *et al.* (2012). Potential association of vitamin D receptor polymorphism Taq1 with multiple sclerosis. *Mult. Scler. J.* **18**, 16–22.

32. Anonymous (2010). Vitamin D: hope on the horizon for MS prevention? *Lancet Neurol.* **9**, 555.

33. Maxmen, A. (2011). Nutrition advice: the vitamin D-lemma. *Nature* **475**, 23–25.

34. Robertson, N.P., Fraser, M., Deans, J., *et al.* (1996). Age-adjusted recurrence risks for relatives of patients with multiple sclerosis. *Brain* **119**, 449–455.

35. Willer, C.J., Dyment, D.A., Risch, N.J., *et al.* (2003). Twin concordance and sibling recurrence rates in multiple sclerosis. *Proc. Natl. Acad. Sci. U.S.A.* **100**, 12877–12882.

36. Olerop, O. and Hillert, J. (1991). HLA class II-associated genetic susceptibility in multiple sclerosis: a critical evaluation. *Tissue Antigens* **38**, 1–15.

37. Lincoln, M.R., Ramagopalan, S.V., Chao, M.J., *et al.* (2009). Epistasis among HLA-DRB1, HLA-DQA1, and HLA-DQB1 loci determines multiple sclerosis susceptibility. *Proc. Natl. Acad. Sci. U.S.A.* **106**, 7542–7547.

38. International Multiple Sclerosis Genetics Consortium (2007). Risk alleles for multiple sclerosis identified by a genomewide study. *N. Engl. J. Med.* **357**, 851–862.

39. Sawcer, S., Hellenthal, G., Pirinen, M., *et al.* (2011). Genetic risk and a primary role for cell-mediated immune mechanisms in multiple sclerosis. *Nature* **476**, 214–219.

40. Costantino, C.M., Baecher-Allan, C., and Hafler, D.A. (2008). Multiple sclerosis and regulatory T cells. *J. Clin. Immunol.* **28**, 697–706.

41. Lucchinetti, C.F., Brück, W., Rodriguez, M., and Lassmann, H. (1996). Distinct patterns of multiple sclerosis pathology indicates heterogeneity on pathogenesis. *Brain Pathol.* **6**, 259–274.

42. Kornek, B. and Lassmann, H. (2003). Neuropathology of multiple sclerosis: new concepts. *Brain Res. Bull.* **61**, 321–326.

Neuropathology of multiple sclerosis

Sandra Amor and Paul van der Valk

Background

Pathology studies of the central nervous system tissues (CNS) from multiple sclerosis (MS) heavily rely on post-mortem tissues obtained from patients with long-standing disease. In rare cases biopsy material is also available when there is suspicion of a tumour allowing study of lesion formation early in the disease. This does not mean, however, that early changes in MS lesion formation cannot be studied and appreciated in autopsy material. Both radiology and pathology have long since shown that new MS lesions develop continuously during the disease process, even after 20 years or more (1, 2, 3). In long-standing disease it is probable that the disease activity changes and this has been associated with a decrease in inflammation in the CNS (4). At this stage the disease becomes more progressive due to the underlying neurodegeneration. Nevertheless, new lesions still form in the very late stages of the disease (5). Therefore, the term 'early MS' should be replaced with 'recently diagnosed' and not associated with a disease in which many new lesions are observed. Rather than a single disease process viewed as a single arching line, pathological changes in MS should be considered a composite of continuously forming small arches, continuing throughout disease until late in the disease course. Each of these lines or small arches runs a pathologically well-characterised course, which has been clearly described (5) and is summarised below. The start of this line we consider to be the pre-active lesion (see below), which develops into the active, then chronic active, and finally chronic inactive lesion. This has been described by many authors and is very applicable to the white matter lesions. The damage observed in the grey matter may be somewhat different (6). How these grey matter lesions develop is not yet clear, simply because they are less inflammatory and the classification of the white matter lesions strongly relies on the evaluation of their inflammatory aspect. Therefore extrapolating findings of white matter lesions to grey matter lesions is difficult. As well as the brain, MS lesions are also observed in the spinal cord, optic nerve, and the deep grey matter regions, including the hippocampus and hypothalamus.

In general, the most consistent aspect of the pathology of MS is its inconsistency in the localisation of lesions, level of inflammation, and extent of demyelination and axonal loss.

Data from pathology have raised questions as to the cause of MS and although autoimmunity almost certainly plays a role in the course of the disease, an autoimmune *cause* for MS has come under some scrutiny. Indeed some demyelinating diseases such as *neuromyelitis optica* may be autoimmune mediated while others result from infections.

The Biology of Multiple Sclerosis, ed Gregory J. Atkins, Sandra Amor, Jean M. Fletcher and Kingston H.G. Mills. Published by Cambridge University Press. © Gregory J. Atkins, Sandra Amor, Jean M. Fletcher and Kingston H.G. Mills 2012.

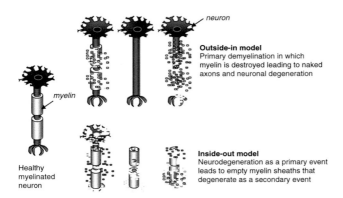

Figure 2.1. Outside-in and inside-out models of demyelination and neuronal damage.

Demyelinating disorders of the CNS

Myelin damage and demyelination of the axons can occur due to a number of pathological mechanisms. Direct damage in which the myelin sheath is lost is termed primary demyelination. In some cases this is also followed by axonal damage and referred to as the outside-in model (Figure 2.1). Alternatively, damage to myelin occurs secondary to axonal damage and neurodegeneration and is termed secondary demyelination, Wallarian degeneration, and more recently, the inside-out model (Figure 2.1).

MS can be classified as an acquired inflammatory demyelinating disorder (Table 2.1). The pathology resembles infectious demyelinating disease and indeed MS is suspected to have viral etiology, but this is still not proven. Interestingly, in the majority of demyelinating disorders of humans and animals in which the etiological agent has been identified, this agent is a virus; for example, progressive multifocal leukoencephalopathy, measles, mumps, and rubella. As well as the classical form of MS, we will briefly discuss the pathology of MS variants.

Hereditary metabolic disorders can be grouped into those in which the onset of damage occurs after the myelin is formed or before myelin is formed leading to hypomyelination (see Table 2.1). In patients with acquired toxic or metabolic disorders such as central pontine myelinolysis, Machiafava–Bignami disease, or vitamin B_{12} deficiency, the lesions of myelin damage are unique and occur in specific regions of the CNS. Finally, myelin damage may also occur due to compression as a result of trauma or a tumour.

History of MS pathology

The first suspected case of MS was reported in a nun, St. Lidwina from Schiedam, The Netherlands in the fourteenth century. Her disease began after a fall while skating, after which she developed clinical signs consistent with MS. These included walking difficulties and vision disturbances interspersed with periods of remission. The clinical and pathological features of MS were first described in detail in the late nineteenth century, although personal accounts and reports of the disease had been noted more than 50 years earlier.

The pioneer Jean Charcot is credited with the full description of the pathology of MS, despite seeing only 34 MS patients during his lifetime. Jean Cruveilhier produced the first

Table 2.1 Characteristics of CNS demyelinating diseases

Group	Disease
Acquired, inflammatory, or infectious	Classical multiple scelrosis
	Relapsing–remitting
	Secondary progressive
	Primary progressive
	Benign
	Variants of multiple scelrosis
	Marburg's type
	Balo's concentric sclerosis
	Schilder's diffuse sclerosis
	Tumefactive MS
	Neuromyelitis optica (Devic's disease)
	Optic neuritis
	Clinically isolated syndrome
	Acute disseminated encephalitis
	Post-infectious encephalomyelitis
	Post-vaccination encephalomyelitis
	Post-immunisation encephalomyelitis
	Acute haemorrhagic leukoencephalopathy
	Progressive multifocal leukoencephalopathy
	Tabes dorsalis
	Transverse myelitis
Hereditary metabolic	Metachromatic leukodystrophy
	Krabbe's disease
	Adrenoleukodystrophy
	Pelizaeus–Merzbacher disease
	Canavan's disease
	Alexander's disease
	Alpers' syndrome (progressive sclerosing poliodystrophy)
	CAMFAK syndrome
Acquired toxic–metabolic	Central pontine myelinolysis
	Machiafava–Bignami disease
	Vitamin B_{12} deficiency
Traumatic	Compression due to extrinsic factors
	Tumour compression

illustrations of the pathology in 1835, although these were not published until several years later. Around the same time Robert Carswell also published his pathological atlas depicting MS lesions, thus predating Cruveilhier by a few years. There is, however, still some controversy regarding who should be credited with its discovery. Carswell studied medicine in Scotland and was commissioned to make illustrations of pathological cases including two cases of MS, which were made while visiting France between 1822–1823 and 1831. Carswell's contemporary Cruveilhier graduated in medicine in Paris in 1811 and went on to attend several patients with '*grise masses disseminées*', the first time the term was used. Several drawings were made of CNS tissues from these patients but the illustrations were not published until 1841. It was not until many years later in 1865 that

Jean Charcot described *sclerose en plaques*, expanding these findings and reports in several papers in the consecutive years. The extent to which Charcot studied MS not only opened the field that laid the foundations of modern research into MS but also led to his recognition as the 'founder' of MS to the extent that MS was actually termed Charcot's disease. Jean Charcot not only recognised that MS was a distinct entity, but also reported the clinical pathological correlations, noting the frequency in the population as well as speculating the pathophysiology. Translation of Charcot's reference to *la sclerose en plaques disseminées* into English gave rise to the term disseminated (cerebrospinal) sclerosis in English speaking countries, while in Germany the term *multiple Sklerose* was used. Since the late nineteenth century many other neuropathologists including Moxon, Hammond, and Rindfleisch, as well as immunologists, virologists, and biochemists, to name just a few disciplines, have greatly added to the knowledge of the pathology of MS. Their findings are discussed in the following sections.

Pathological subtypes of MS

The recognition of other clinical forms of MS, such as where the spinal cord is severely affected, was already noted by Charcot. Here we discuss the pathology of these subtypes and classical forms of MS as well as several closely associated inflammatory demyelinating disorders.

Marburg's disease

Marburg's fulminant MS is also referred to as acute MS. It was first recognised by Otto Marburg in 1909, and manifest by rapid deterioration in the clinical condition reflected by changes observed by MRI examination. Patients present with a rapid development and progression of multiple demyelinating lesions that do not respond well to conventional treatments. Eventually patients with Marburg's MS develop a persistent coma and tetraparesis within several months to a year from first symptoms. Death is mainly related to brainstem involvement. Pathologically, the lesions are much more destructive than classical MS and contain many regions of macrophage infiltration, acute axonal injury, and necrosis (7).

Balo's concentric sclerosis

This form of MS was first recorded by Joseph Balo in 1927. Patients with Balo's MS present with an acute fulminant disease that progress rapidly to death within months. The pathology is characterised by a unique pattern of concentric demyelination in the CNS that resembles onion bulbs. This pattern is also seen in imaging studies that reveal alternating concentric hyperintense rings that may enhance with gadolinium. Several reports describe these lesions in other forms of MS and acute disseminated encephalomyelitis (ADEM –see below).

Neuromyelitis optica

Neuromyelitis optica (NMO) also known as Devic's disease, is an inflammatory demyelinating condition generally affecting the optic nerves and spinal cord in which longitudinal extensive transverse myelitis is observed. In some cases lesions are also present in the brain and in children with NMO basal ganglia and hypothalamic lesions are observed. These demyelinated plaques in NMO show little evidence of remyelination. Based on the lesion distribution as well as the immunology, NMO is considered distinct from MS since the damage in NMO is associated with the presence of autoantibodies to the astrocytic water channel aquaporin 4 (AQP4) (8). These antibodies are diagnostic of disease and are pathogenic as shown by their effect when injected into animals.

Schilder's disease

This form of MS is also referred to as Schilder's diffuse sclerosis, or myelinoclastic diffuse sclerosis. It is a rare demyelinating disease first identified by Paul Schilder in 1912 in a 14-year-old girl. Typically Schilder's disease is manifested by rapid decline in mental function often associated with increased intracranial pressure and leading to death within months. It is more often seen in children although adult onset has also been reported. The pathology is typically characterised by bilateral, large hemispheric demyelinating lesions measuring at least 3 x 2 cm in the centrum semiovale of the cerebral hemispheres with histological characteristics identical to MS. The lesions of demyelination may be focal as in MS or more diffuse; and active demyelination is associated with inflammation. In some cases, however, single lesions are reported and in one case optic neuritis was observed in addition to lesions in the cerebral hemispheres (9). The close similarities with other demyelinating diseases such as ADEM and classical MS have provoked reviews of the reported cases in which 70% were diagnosed as MS (10).There is no data on the gender bias in these forms of MS.

Tumefactive MS

Large rapidly expanding lesions in the brain suggestive of a tumour such as gliomas or metastases or multiple cysts are seen in some forms of MS. These lesions are not tumours but rapidly expanding demyelinating lesions. A review of cases of pathologically confirmed tumefactive demyelinating lesions showed that most were part of a clinical and/or radiological picture consistent with MS (11, 12). Following diagnosis of a demyelinating condition the patients improved with corticosteroid therapy. No cases were suggestive of Schilder's or Balo's concentric sclerosis. The pathology of tumefactive MS is reminiscent of acute MS in which foamy lipid laden macrophages and activated microglia are observed alongside areas of myelin loss. Tumefactive MS is characterised by lesions > 2 cm with oedema and/or ring enhancement at MRI.

Two other acquired inflammatory demyelinating diseases deserve mention. These are acute disseminated encephalomyelitis and acute haemorrhagic leukoencephalopathy, both of which are reminiscent of MS and important to consider in the differential diagnosis.

Acute disseminated encephalomyelitis

Acute disseminated encephalomyelitis (ADEM) is generally monophasic although in rare cases relapsing forms have been reported, and occurs with a temporal and probably also a causative relationship to a viral infection (post-infection encephalomyelitis), as well as to vaccination (post-vaccination encephalomyelitis) (13). Like MS, ADEM is characterised by inflammation and demyelination in the brain and spinal cord, but is distinguished by the perivenous localisation of the pathological changes and thus is also known as a perivenous encephalomyelitis. In addition to the inflammation, large areas of demyelination are also reported. Inflammation is observed in the cortical regions as well as white matter and is especially pronounced perivenously. Inflammation is composed of T cells, B cells, and plasma cells coinciding with demyelination around the blood vessels. Like MS, lipid laden macrophages are observed in the demyelinated areas, occurring together with degrees of axonal damage. In acute ADEM, haemorrhages are observed around blood vessels and in some cases fibrin deposits are present in vessel walls.

Acute haemorrhagic leukoencephalopathy

Acute haemorrhagic leukoencephalopathy (AHL) is more aggressive and has a higher morbidity and mortality than ADEM. Like ADEM, AHL is associated with viral infections and although this disease is generally monophasic, relapsing forms have been described. Lesions in the CNS are typically inflammatory, haemorrhagic, and demyelinating. Studies reporting AHL are rare and thus it is difficult to determine gender bias. In one study of 30 patients with post-infectious perivenous encephalitis, 26 were male and 4 female while in a study of 8 AHL patients, 6 were male and 2 female.

Multiple sclerosis

Classical MS subtypes are classified by clinical features. Approximately 85% of people present with relapsing–remitting episodes of neurological deficits – so-called relapsing–remitting MS (RRMS). In some RRMS cases a gradual increase in the neurological deficits occurs and the disease becomes progressive; a stage referred to as secondary progressive MS (SPMS). In approximately 15% of cases the disease is progressive from the onset with only minor improvements or plateaus in disease. Except in cases where lesions arise in vital areas, or in the case of biopsies (as in tumefactive MS – see above), the majority of pathological tissues collected in MS tissue banks come from patients with either primary progressive MS (PPMS) or secondary progressive stage. The detailed pathology is discussed in detail later in the chapter.

MS: gross pathology

Pathological examination of the brain and spinal cord from chronic MS patients may reveal greyish plaques or lesions on the surface of the optic nerve, chiasm, brainstem, and spinal cord. In severe chronic cases atrophy of the brain and spinal cord is observed and the brain weight may be reduced. All regions of the CNS can be affected by MS although there is a predilection for certain sites.

Dissection of the brain reveals greyish shrunken lesions that are often fibrous due to astrogliosis of chronic inactive lesions. These are frequently observed around the ventricles and clearly identifiable in the white matter, often associated with blood vessels. The proclivity for lesions around blood vessels was first documented by Dawson giving rise to the term 'Dawson's fingers' (14).

With the focus on grey matter pathology, careful examination of the brain also reveals lesions within the cortical regions. These grey matter lesions are far less obvious than white matter lesions and this is probably the reason for MS being originally considered a purely white matter disease. Thus MS should be thought as both a grey and white matter disease, where the grey matter pathology plays a key role in cognitive disability. As will be explained later, lesion development does not respect borders and so-called type 1 grey matter lesions are in fact areas where the lesion has expanded into both the white and grey

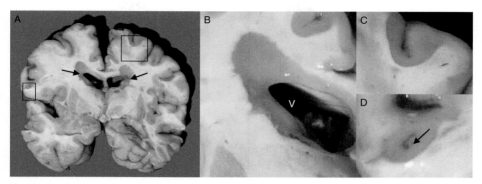

Figure 2.2. Gross pathology of MS. (A) Saggital section of the brain showing typical periventricular lesions (arrows) in MS and enlarged in (B) (v – ventricle). Boxes in (A) outline two other lesions (C) and (D). (C) is clearly a grey matter lesion impinging on a clearly demarcated lesion edge while lesion (D) centres on a blood vessel (arrow). See plate section for colour version.

matter. As well as the gross pathology, post-mortem magnetic resonance imaging (MRI) of the MS brain reveals many more lesions than observed with the naked eye.

Distribution of lesions

While MS lesions can arise anywhere in the CNS they show a predilection for several areas including the optic nerve, spinal cord, and brainstem. In addition, tissues adjacent to the ventricles (Figure 2.2), subarachnoid space, and the aqueduct of Sylvius are especially vulnerable to demyelination suggesting that soluble toxic factors in the CSF may play a role in tissue damage. While spinal cord atrophy provides the best correlation with progressive disability there is no regularity regarding the distribution of lesions. Intriguingly, the lesions in the spinal cord and optic nerve show the most chronic changes, which may be due to several factors including differences in the blood–tissue barrier in these locations. More recently studies have also revealed evidence of retinal atrophy, retinal ganglion cell loss, axonal loss, and injury as well as neuronal loss associated with HLA-DR positive microglia. In addition injury to both iris and retina could be seen at all stages of disease. These later studies may explain the studies showing reduced retinal ganglion cell layer using optical coherence tomography (15).

Histopathology

As mentioned above MS pathology is generally focussed on the study of tissues from patients with long-standing or established MS. However, the availability of early active lesions, derived from patients dying early in disease or from biopsy tissues obtained from patients presenting with a tumour-like lesion, has allowed insight into pathology in early disease. The study of early MS led to the classification of four patterns of lesions assumed to be due to heterogeneous mechanisms of demyelination (16) (Table 2.2). In contrast, a study of established MS, i.e. after long disease duration, revealed a homogeneous pattern in which immunoglobulin and complement deposits were observed (17) (see Table 2.2).

Table 2.2 The heterogeneous and homogeneous views of MS pathology

Pattern	Characteristics
Heterogeneous view	
I	Macrophage and T cell immune pattern without complement deposition
II	Deposition of antibodies and C9neo on damaged myelin sheaths and oligodendrocytes. Occasional apoptosis
III	Oligodendrogliopathy. Oligodendrocyte apoptosis with a preferential early and substantial loss of myelin-associated glycoprotein (MAG)
IV	Non-apoptotic degeneration of oligodendrocytes. Subtype found in a few primary progressive cases
Homogeneous view	
II	Immunoglobulin and complement deposits in 100% established MS cases

Demyelination

As discussed above myelin damage may be due to direct attack (outside-in model) or follow axonal damage and wallerian degeneration (inside-out model). In MS both naked axons and so-called empty myelin sheaths are observed indicating both mechanisms are operational. Interestingly there is preferential loss of myelin on thin calibre axons. That antibodies and complement contribute to myelin damage is reflected by the pattern II lesion described by Lucchinetti and colleagues (16) and observed in established MS lesions (17). In animal models antibodies to myelin protein augment disease-inducing myelin damage. Demyelination in MS is associated with so-called foamy macrophages that have taken up myelin. In vitro studies reveal a temporal sequence of myelin degradation with minor myelin proteins, such as myelin oligodendrocyte glycoprotein and the myelin-associated small heat-shock protein alpha B crystallin, being degraded first (18). Neutral lipids remain in the macrophage lysosomes and are oil-red O and periodic acid Schiff reaction positive (Figure 2.3). This is the active MS lesion. In some cases nearby blood vessels show tissue infiltration by T cells and B cells (see Figure 2.3) together with activated microglia and macrophages. Demyelination progresses centrifugally giving rise to the chronic active lesion with foam cells at the rim of the lesion. In addition so-called diffusely/dirty appearing white matter shows large areas of disrupted myelin (19) associated with activated microglia. As explained below, prior to the active lesion and at the point of lesion expansion is the so-called pre-active lesion in which myelin is intact.

Remyelination

As a consequence of the myelin damage, oligodendrocyte progenitors repopulate the damaged area allowing remyelination. Such areas are observed in EM studies as thinly myelinated axons which have shorter internodes and present at the periphery of lesions as well as within the white matter. Areas of remyelination, observed as clearly demarcated regions of pale myelin (Figure 2.3), are referred to as shadow plaques. Significantly more remyelination is observed in early lesions than in chronic MS (80.7% versus 60%) (20). Intriguingly in chronic MS, subcortical lesions were reported to show more extensive

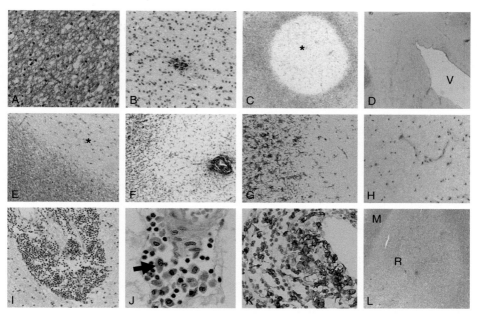

Figure 2.3. Pathology of MS. (A) Normal appearing white matter stained with luxol fast blue in MS frequently contains clusters of HLA class II positive macrophages that cluster to form a pre-active lesion (B, brown HLA class II immunohistochemistry). (C) MBP staining for myelin (brown) shows a chronic active lesion the centre of which is devoid of myelin (*). (D) A periventricular lesion (V = ventricle) showing a large area of demyelination, LFB stain. In (E) the edge of the lesion is clearly demarcated showing normal appearing myelin (LFB stain) with the demyelinated centre (*). (F) HLA class II positive cells at the rim of a chronic active lesion and perivascular. (G) High power. (H) Centre of inactive lesion is hypocellular and devoid of myelin. (I) A large perivascular cuff of T cells, B cells, and macrophages. (J) Higher power showing some of these cells are foamy macrophages that have engulfed myelin (arrow). A high proportion of these infiltrates are B cells (brown) K. (L) A shadow plaque (pale blue area – R) surrounded by normal appearing myelin, M, representing an area of remyelination. See plate section for colour version.

remyelination than periventricular lesions (21). Remyelination correlates with the presence of high numbers of oligodendrocytes expressing myelin proteins or myelin protein mRNA in their cytoplasm, and the expression of developmental genes by oligodendrocytes, as well as an increased expression of bcl-2 – a cell death inhibitory protein. As already mentioned characteristics of remyelination are best recognised using electron microscopy and have mainly been defined in the toxin-induced cuprizone model. Recently detailed transcriptomic analysis in this model reveals a microglia phenotype that supports remyelination already at the onset of demyelination and persists throughout the remyelination process (22). While this has yet to be examined in MS these microglia express a cytokine and chemokine repertoire enabling activation and recruit of endogenous oligodendrocyte progenitor cells to the lesion site. As well as microglia, activated astrocytes may play a role in endogenous repair processes. Again in the cuprizone model, studies have revealed a possible role for the radial-glial cell marker brain lipid binding protein (BLBP, FABP7) that correlates with the presence of oligodendrocyte progenitor cells. BLBP-expressing astrocytes are present in early MS lesions and less so in patients with long disease duration (23).

Neurodegeneration and axonal damage

As mentioned already axonal damage is a major component of the pathology of MS. It is observed in the demyelinating plaques and also in the normal appearing white matter (NAWM). As stressed above axonal damage and neurodegeneration could occur due to the absence of trophic support by myelin during myelin destruction. In ongoing demyelinating areas particularly in the active plaque and at the edge of chronic active lesions activated microglia and macrophages are known to produce a plethora of potentially damaging compounds, thus contributing to both myelin and axonal damage. It is these regions where axonal bulbs reflecting transsected or damaged axons may undergo phagocytosis (24). Furthermore, there is evidence that axons in normal appearing white matter also undergo degeneration. One explanation is that wallerian degeneration in periplaque regions (25) leads to pathology distant from the lesion. Similarly, neuronal loss is also observed in both the affected demyelinated grey matter as well as the normal appearing grey matter (NAGM). Thus while damage occurs in the microscopically visible lesions, diffuse changes also occur distant from these lesions.

Oligodendrocyte damage

In chronic MS lesions, low numbers of immature Galactocerebroside (GalC)-positive oligodendrocytes are present together with low numbers of oligodendrocyte precursor cells (OPCs) consistent with the failure of myelin repair in late stages of MS. In contrast, in recently demyelinated areas mature oligodendrocytes express GalC and MOG (a marker for mature oligodendrocytes) suggesting that these cells have survived the loss of myelin. In these areas large numbers of cells are observed throughout the lesion and at the edges of older lesions. Demyelinated oligodendrocytes are more frequent in areas with macrophages than areas lacking macrophages (26). Thus, two principal patterns of oligodendrocyte pathology have been reported; the proliferation in remyelinated areas as discussed above and damage during active demyelination. While the exact mechanism of cell damage and death is still under debate oligodendrocytes are known to be susceptible to damage via a number of immune or toxic mechanisms. Such damage involves the cytokines such as TNFα or IFN-γ, ROS and NOS, glutamate, complement, and lytic enzymes, all components present in MS lesions. Specific injury could occur due to T cell-mediated damage, Fas-Fas-ligand interactions or CD8[+] mediated cytotoxicity. Lastly, persistent viral infection may also play a role.

Oligodendrocytes in MS express TNF-R1 and TNF-R2, and their expression levels are influenced by factors such as age or neurodegenerative damage. In the pre-phagocytic periplaque regions, oligodendrocytes bear markers of apoptosis (27) while pre-active lesions express markers such as alpha B crystallin, a heat-shock protein, production of which is suggested to be an attempt to resist apoptosis (28).

Astrocytes

Despite the early suggestions by Muller that MS was a disease of astrocytes, the role of astrocytes in MS has generally been considered to be in the formation of the gliotic scar, present in inactive lesions. However, astrocytes play a key role in the maintenance of the blood and spinal cord barrier as well as having a dual role in aiding degeneration by promoting inflammation, but also in allowing remyelination by their action on oligodendrocyte precursors and differentiation.

In early MS lesions, changes in the level of astrocytes are observed. The cells become hypertrophic and may contain fragmented nuclei. In the lesion and surrounding tissues these cells express unregulated glial fibrillary acid protein (GFAP) as well as vimentin and re-express nestin. In the ongoing demyelinated plaque, astrocytes are the most abundant cell type expressing matrix metalloproteinases (MMP) (29), which may be involved in tissue damage or alternatively in tissue remodelling. Astrocytes also express chemokines and cytokines in active and chronic active lesions, including monocyte chemoattractant factor, tumour necrosis factor alpha (TNFα) (30), nitric oxide synthase (NOS) (31), CXCL12, and B cell activating factor (BAFF;32), thus aiding recruitment of macrophages and B cells and contributing to tissue damage (for review see 33).

Alternatively, astrocytes have also been implicated in remyelination, as a result of their expression of chemoattractant molecules (CXCL1, CXCL8, and CXCL10), semaphorins, aiding the recruitment of oligodendrocyte progenitor cells. The expression of fibroblast growth factor-2 within activated astrocytes in MS lesions could aid oligodendrocyte progenitor cell proliferation while expression of excitatory amino acid transporters could help cell survival by limiting glutamate toxicity. Finally astrocytes in MS may play a role in oligodendrocyte differentiation and maturation in MS lesions, since studies have reported expression of ciliary neurotrophic factor (CNTF) and interleukin (IL)-11 known to promote differentiation of mature oligodendrocytes in vitro (34).

Mitochondrial damage

Mechanisms involved in lesion formation include oxidative damage (for review see 35). Several studies show the abundance of oxidised lipids, proteins, and DNA in active MS lesions. Lipid peroxides and oxidised nuclear DNA were detected in oligodendrocytes as well as in axonal bulbs and degenerating neurons and to a lesser extent in astrocytes (36). The presence of oxidised lipids is not surprising given the levels of macrophage and microglia activation in MS lesions and thus high levels of reactive oxygen and nitrogen species. However, the periplaque white matter around the developing lesions was found to contain significant oxidative stress probably as a result of macrophage, microglia, and astrocyte reactivity. The presence of damage in the periplaque white matter suggests that T cells do not play a major role in the initiation of this damage. Mitochondrial pathology is the earliest ultrastructural sign of damage in the CNS and while it precedes changes in axon morphology, this stage is reversible (37). Mitochondria increase within axons as a result of demyelination as a response to changes in energy requirements due to redistribution of sodium channels; however, enhanced density of mitochondria in MS lesions might contribute to the formation of free radicals and exacerbate ongoing tissue damage.

Stress proteins

Under stress conditions, such as in the presence of inflammatory mediators, reduced oxygen or infections, cells respond by producing so-called 'stress' or 'heat-shock' proteins (HSPs). HSPs are stress-induced chaperones important in preventing protein misfolding and inhibiting apoptotic activity and thus are thought to play a protective role in neurodegenerative diseases including MS. Expression of different HSPs has been reported in MS (Table 2.3). In Balo's concentric sclerosis where high expression of inducible NOS was

Table 2.3 Heat-shock protein expression in MS CNS

HSP	Presence	Reference
αB crystallin (HSPB5)	In oligodendrocytes in pre-active and active lesions, and in hypertrophic astrocytes	38 28
HSP27 (HSPB1)	Increased 2.5–4 fold in lesions, in astrocytes and oligodendrocytes at lesion edge	39
HSP32 (HO-1)	In oligodendrocytes in early MS lesions and in microglia/ macrophages and astrocytes in ADEM	40
HSP60	In corpora amylacea bodies	41
HSP65	Expression in cytoplasm of MBP+ immature oligodendrocytes as well as astrocytes, microglia, and endothelial cells	42 43
HSP70	Stress-induced. No difference in expression between normal and MS white matter	39
HSC70	73 kDa constitutive expression. Reduced expression in MS lesions. 30–50% reduction compared to control myelin as assessed by immunoblotting	39

found in macrophages and microglia, hypoxia-inducible factor 1α and HSP70 were expressed in oligodendrocytes (44). The role of HSPs in regulating and controlling apoptosis may explain the expression of HSPs in oligodendrocytes in MS lesions. HSPs can be secreted from cells, and for the small HSPs αB crystallin may play a role in microglia activation in early MS lesions (28,45,46).

Lesion staging and evolution
White matter lesions

MS is generally considered a white matter disease for understandable reasons, as most myelin is found in white matter, but research has brought to light that there are also important abnormalities in the grey matter. However, the grey matter pathology is much more subtle (see below) and many of our insights in MS come from studies of white matter pathology, especially where the time frame of the disease is considered, next to, of course, the cells involved in the process. Thus, careful studies have suggested a certain sequence of events leading to the formation of a scar-like lesion, the well-known grey, hard, sclerotic lesion that gave the disease its name. Earlier lesions show a solid and hypercellular lesion, composed primarily of phagocytising macrophages, filled with myelin debris and its breakdown products. Gradually this lesion dies out in the centre leaving a scar-like lesion with a rim of remaining phagocytes, only to die out completely leaving a gliotic scar, hypocellular and devoid of myelin. Data from MRI studies suggest that this process takes weeks to months to complete. One of the unanswered questions is what precedes the active lesions (solid macrophages) and we have suggested that there is a lesion in which there is no demyelination yet, but that does show activation of microglia, the so-called pre-active lesion, that may very well be the first visible manifestation of MS in the tissue.

The pre-active lesion

As stated above, a pre-active lesion is a cluster of activated (HLA-DR expressing) microglia in an area of 'normal' myelin. These lesions are not always associated with vessels, indicating that the inciting event probably comes from the CNS tissue itself and not necessarily from the blood. An occasional lymphocyte can be found in or next to a vessel in the vicinity of pre-active lesions, but otherwise there are no abnormalities visible in the tissue. There are no detectable levels of complement or immunoglobulin deposition, no demonstrable blood–brain barrier (BBB) dysfunction (47), and no depletion of oligodendrocytes in grey matter lesions. However, immunohistochemical studies demonstrate that the oligodendrocytes are stressed, i.e. they express the HSP αB crystallin (28). Most of these lesions are found in the vicinity of active and chronic active lesions, and less frequently near inactive lesions. Of course, microglial activation is not a particularly specific phenomenon and is also seen in areas of remyelination or the so-called diffusely abnormal white matter (48,49), but the tight clustering is fairly typical for what we call pre-active lesions. Occasionally, a lesion is found where a rare foamy macrophage is present among the microglia and myelin is beginning to degenerate, suggesting transition to an active lesion.

The fascinating aspect of these lesions is that they can be numerous at any point in disease progression, suggesting that not all of these lesions will progress to an active lesion; apparently the brain has the ability to regress these lesions, thus preventing formation of an active lesion and, at times, a scar. It is not known how the brain tissue controls this damage limitation, but elucidation of this process would open the way to switching off lesion formation.

The active lesion

At a critical point myelin damage will elicit an inflammatory response and macrophages are recruited by bringing in monocytes from the blood. What triggers this is unknown, but findings in grey matter lesions, where myelin is scanty and inflammatory responses rare, suggest that the amount of myelin might be crucial to determining the severity of the inflammation. It has been pointed out that this is not just detrimental but the clearance of myelin debris is an important factor in allowing remyelination to occur. So the macrophage can be friend, foe, or maybe even both.

Amongst this mass of macrophages that characterises the active lesion oligodendrocytes can also be seen in increased, decreased, or normal numbers. Some investigators have indicated that apoptosis of oligodendrocytes is a very attractive explanation for the eventual loss of these cells. However, we were unable to corroborate this, since while nuclear condensation was fairly frequent, nuclear fragmentation, the inevitable next step in apoptosis, was not observed (van der Valk, unpublished data). Astrocytes are also present within active lesions, showing hypertrophy with an increased amount of cytoplasm and numbers of protrusions.

The amount of axonal damage in active lesions is a matter of debate. That some degree of damage will occur in a battlefield that an active lesion represents is perhaps not surprising. In a seminal paper by Dutta and Trapp (50) the number of axonal bulbs, assuming that an axonal bulb represents axonal transsection, was analysed. This study revealed huge numbers of bulbs, indicating extensive neuronal damage early in lesion formation. Whether a bulb truly represents an axonal transsection in all cases is not certain and the fact that neurological deficit can disappear in this relapsing–remitting disease suggests that not all damage is permanent. Unfortunately, there is no other validated study reporting on axonal damage other than counting bulbs. More research is necessary in this area.

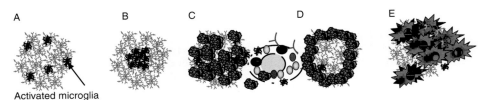

Figure 2.4. Lesion progression in MS. Normal appearing white matter in MS (A) with occasional activated microglia. In the pre-active lesion, microglia migrate and form a cluster (B). An unknown trigger recruits macrophages from the blood and these cells phagocytose myelin – red globules inside the cells in an active lesion (C) and at the rim of a chronic active lesion (D). The centre of an inactive lesion is composed of hypertrophic astrocytes – the gliotic scar (E). See plate section for colour version.

In active lesions, lymphocytes are predominantly present in the perivascular space, where they form cuffs around the blood vessels. The number of lymphocytes in the parenchyma is limited in most cases. Immunohistochemistry reveals that of the T cells, CD8+ cells may predominate over CD4+ T cells in the earlier stages, but T cells outnumber B cells in most cases. However, the number of B cells in the perivascular space and in the meninges is a somewhat controversial issue. Mostly their number is limited to perivascular regions with very few in the meninges. Reports on conglomerates of B cells (follicle-like structures) (51) have not been reproduced in different centres (52). Whether technical concerns can explain these differences or whether this can be attributed to differences in patient groups is not certain (53). In our experience B cell aggregates are very rare, irrespective of the location (perivascular cuffs, meninges in the sulci, surface meninges) and follicular structures are not seen.

The chronic active lesion

This stage is a logical progression of the active lesion. At the centre of the lesion myelin is completely absent following clearance by macrophages. After phagocytosis the foamy macrophages have no more reason to be there and they leave, probably by route of the perivascular spaces. In sections foamy macrophages are observed at the edge of the demyelinated centre and may also be seen clustering in the perivascular space. Foamy macrophages containing myelin and neuronal debris are also observed in the cerebrospinal fluid (24). In the centre the oligodendrocytes are diminished and astrogliosis is seen, with some hypertrophic astrocytes. In time, the number of phagocytising macrophages in the rim decreases and the lesion dies out.

The chronic inactive lesion

This is the typical grey, sunken, sclerotic lesion seen upon macroscopy. It is a demyelinated area, hypocellular throughout, densely gliotic, with typical isomorphic gliosis. The few cells are mostly astrocytes; oligodendrocytes are virtually absent. Some remaining macrophages and perivascular lymphocytes can persist for quite some time, but overall the impression is of low cellularity (Figure 2.4E).

The proposed development of the MS lesion is shown in Figure 2.4; it can occur almost everywhere in the CNS and during the disease lesions like this spring up, run their course, and turn to scars, probably in a continuous fashion, until the inflammatory components die out and the neurodegenerative aspect takes full swing, leading the patient into the secondary progressive phase. Even after many years of disease one can see this process still occurring.

One of the more mysterious aspects of this process is the phenomenon of synchronisation, i.e. the fact that in a given patient lesions tend to be at the same stage. If the occurrence of new lesions is random in time and the process always runs the same course, then one should see all lesional stages similarly represented (maybe with predominance of the stage that lasts the longest). However, this is not the case; there is synchronisation although it is uncertain how such synchronisation occurs.

There are additional pathological changes observed in MS tissues including remyelination as discussed above. Sharply demarcated areas of decreased intensity of myelin staining (especially in luxol fast blue stains), the so-called shadow plaques, are considered to represent remyelination. This is largely based on electron microscopical studies in experimental systems showing that remyelinated axons have thinner myelin sheaths (and shorter internodes); less myelin means less myelin staining in a stochastic dye such as luxol fast blue, so these shadow plaques are good candidates for areas of remyelination. In our experience, it is not really possible to see in a paraffin section that myelin sheaths are thinner. Alternative explanations for the diminished staining could be any loss of axons, or any decrease in axonal density (oedema), or even partial demyelination.

Periplaque white matter

As discussed above oxidative stress reflected by the presence of oxidised lipids and DNA is highly pronounced in the periplaque white matter surrounding the actively expanding MS lesion (36). This region has also been termed pre-phagocytic (27) and may be comparable to the pre-active lesion discussed above although comparative studies have not been performed. Earlier studies revealed that molecular changes are present in the periplaque areas. Here genes involved in protection against oxidative stress – haemoxygenase-1–were increased concomitantly with the presence of neuronal NOS suggesting intrinsic mechanisms are in place to facilitate protection (54).

Cortical grey matter pathology

Though the first reports on grey matter pathology date from 1916 these findings were ignored until the 1990s. The axiom that MS was a white matter disorder was brutally dominant. To some extent this was due to technical reasons. It was not until the last two decades of the last century that immunohistochemical staining of myelin became widely applied. Before that, evaluation of myelin was done by luxol fast blue staining. Staining of grey matter in luxol fast blue is minimal because myelin is present in small amounts, making any loss of myelin difficult to appreciate. With immunohistochemical stains for myelin proteins minor changes are more easily detected and grey matter demyelination has been shown to be very common in MS and often quite widespread. Another reason that cortical pathology had gone undetected for so long became apparent: there is virtually no inflammatory reaction, defined by the presence of macrophages and/or lymphocytes in or around areas of demyelination in the grey matter, at least in established disease. In addition to documenting the presence of demyelination, some typical patterns were seen. This led to the description of four types of grey matter lesions (55) (Figure 2.5).

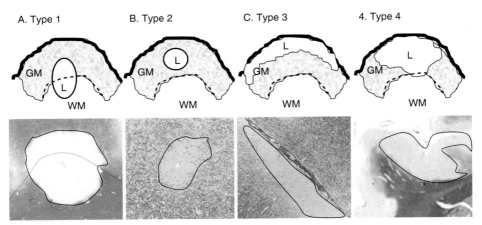

Figure 2.5. Diagrammatic representation of grey matter lesions. The representations above are diagrams showing the different grey matter lesions that depict the lesions observed in MS below. The meninges are depicted as a continuous thick black line, the edge of the lesion as a thin black line, and the border of the white and grey matter as a dotted line. GM, grey matter; WM, white matter; L demyelinated lesions. See plate section for colour version.

The type 1 lesion

The type 1 (leucocorticoid) lesion (see Figure 2.5A) is a combined grey and white matter lesion. The proportion of the white and grey matter parts is variable, but they usually form a clear roundish lesion that simply ignores the grey-white matter boundary. This is of some importance as in many instances the white matter part shows some activity (i.e. at least chronic active or active stage), while the grey matter part shows no activity, despite the topography of the lesion strongly suggesting it concerns one lesion. The lack of inflammation in the grey matter part is unlikely to be due to the lesion being old and exhausted. It is more likely to be due to the fact that local factors in the grey matter have an immunosuppressive effect. Thus, the white matter part of a type 1 lesion shows an area of demyelination and inflammatory changes, whereas the grey matter part shows no changes besides the demyelination. There are no activated macrophages, no lymphocytes, no depositions of complement or immunoglobulin, and no BBB dysfunction (47). In some cases an incomplete rim of activated microglia extends from the edge of the white matter part into the grey matter, suggesting part of the border of the lesion, but foam cells are not seen.

The type 2 lesion

This is an entirely intracortical area of demyelination (see Figure 2.5B), similar to the grey matter part of a type 1 lesion, that is demyelinated but devoid of inflammatory cells.

The type 3 lesion

This is an extremely interesting pattern in which the area directly below the leptomeningeal covering (i.e. layers I, II, and III predominantly, but it can extend deeper) is stripped of myelin (see Figure 2.5C). These lesions can be very extensive and not infrequently almost the entire surface of the brain can be involved. Histologically, they are similar to type 2 lesions, i.e. demyelinated and non-inflammatory. With the presence of the neuronal cell bodies in the immediate vicinity it is probable that such myelin loss will have clinical implications. The distribution, so close to the cerebrospinal fluid (CSF), suggests that something in the CSF may be causative. So far, however, the clinical impact has not been clearly demonstrated and the toxic agent in the CSF that could be responsible for type 3 lesions is unknown.

The type 4 lesion

This is a cortical lesion that involves the entire cortical width (see Figure 2.5D). It is not clear whether this is a distinct entity. Some type 3 lesions extend deeper to involve the entire cortical width and it is conceivable that an enlarging type 2 lesion will eventually become a type 4 lesion. Histologically the type 4 lesions are indistinguishable from the other types.

Deep grey matter

The cortical lesions in most instances respect the grey-white matter border (apart from the type 1 lesions). This is somewhat different in the deep grey matter and in the spinal cord (see below). Lesions in the deep grey matter often do not respect the grey-white matter border. They often show larger lesions extensively involving both the grey matter and the white matter areas around it. This is clearly demonstrated in studies of the hippocampus and in the hypothalamus in MS. Similar to the cortical lesion the lesions are non-inflammatory and often microglial activation is seen in areas of remaining myelin, but not in the grey matter lesions themselves.

Spinal cord

Similar to the brain the lesions in the spinal cord are often extensive and frequently involve both grey and white matter. Compared to brain lesions most MS lesions in the spinal cord resemble old lesions, with little inflammatory activity, even lesions entirely located in the white matter. In these areas a great number of swollen axons reflect extensive axonal damage leading to loss of up to 70% of axons compared to a non-lesional area in the contralateral side of the cord. Regarding neuronal loss both motor neurons and interneurons are reduced in MS at the cervical and thoracic but not lumbar levels (56). This study showed that motor neuron loss was predominantly related to nearby grey matter lesions, whereas interneuron loss was observed in both myelinated and demyelinated areas.

Macrophage accumulations in lesions are not as compact as active lesions in the brain; the infiltrates are more dispersed and less densely packed. In the spinal cord one can also see areas of decreased intensity of myelin staining. Some of these areas could be due to wallerian degeneration, or to remyelination, and are not as sharply defined as shadow plaques in the brain.

The meninges

The meningeal compartment is not strictly behind the BBB and therefore would allow for easy antigen uptake and thus antigen processing and initiation of immune responses. In light of this, the description of myelin/myelin remnants in the meninges is of considerable interest (57). In addition, inflammatory infiltrates can be found in the meninges, apparently unrelated to the presence or absence of underlying grey or white matter lesions; however, this is still controversial as some reports show that grey matter damage is directly related to inflammation in the meninges (58). As in the perivascular cuffs, the predominant cell type is the T-lymphocyte, but macrophages and small numbers of dendritic cells and B cells are also present. As mentioned before another controversial issue is the detection of ectopic B cell follicles thought to be related to EBV infection (51). The significance of these findings is not yet clear but could be the underlying reason for the oligoclonal immunoglobulin bands present in the CSF in MS.

Inflammation

Despite the immune-privileged nature of the CNS both innate and adaptive immune responses are observed in the MS brain indicting that either such responses are initiated within the CNS behind a closed BBB or that during disease the BBB is compromised. The innate immune system is the first line of defence, to opsonise and clear apoptotic cells and infections. A second crucial step is to recruit the adaptive immune responses including cytokines and chemokines that induce adhesion molecules on the BBB and co-stimulatory molecules on microglia. Inflammation is considered to be a key event in the initiation of MS and there is an association between inflammation and neurodegeneration in all lesions and disease stages. However, inflammation in the CNS may die out in patients with long-standing disease since the level of inflammation is similar to that observed in age-matched controls (59). In our experience, some MS patients, despite long-standing disease, do show increased inflammation associated with chronic active lesions and perivascular cuffs that are not due to confounding pathologies.

Innate immunity

Although early studies in MS focussed on T cells and antibodies, assuming a role for autoimmune T and B cells in MS, there is currently a general awareness that through conserved pattern recognition receptors, local CNS cells may be triggered to develop innate responses. Among the innate receptors are toll-like receptors (TLRs) (60), C type lectins, and NOD-like receptors (NLR), although, apart from TLR, little is known about their expression in the activation of microglia or indeed astrocytes in MS. These receptors bind pathogen-associated molecular patterns (PAMPs) or damaged or stressed tissues (danger-associated molecular patterns, or DAMPs). DAMPs present in MS tissues include heat-shock proteins, uric acid, chromatin, adenosine and ATP, and high mobility group box chromosomal protein-1 (HMGB-1), galectins and thioredoxin (for review see 61). Also a reflection of innate immunity in MS lesions are components of the inflammasome, a multiprotein complex known to activate caspase-1 (62) and -5 and trigger production of IL-1β, IL-18, and IL-33. Inflammasome assembly relies on NOD-like receptor family members and interaction with TLRs. As well as innate receptors, the complement system and several cytokines associated with the innate immune system, including IL-6, IL-1β, TNFα, and type I interferons (IFNs), are present in MS lesions (28, 63). Evidence that the complete system is activated in MS is reflected by several reports showing complement components in demyelinating lesions. For example C3, membrane attack complex (MAC), and immunoglobulin deposits have been reported in areas of demyelination (64, 65). Complement C3 and Ig complexes are present on basement membranes and also in the pre-phagocytic regions surrounding active and chronic active lesions (66). The presence of complement and immunoglobulins has been used to classify different types of pathology in MS (16) although this is still controversial (17).

Microglia and macrophages

The presence of activated microglia and macrophages within MS lesions is clear evidence of innate immune activation (45, 67). The activation state and stage of degradation of myelin inside macrophages within lesions are considered useful for staging the early lesions of MS. Indeed clusters of activated microglia in normal appearing white matter typify the pre-active lesion, while foamy macrophages are characteristic of both the active and chronic active lesions. Although microglia play an important role in the pathology of MS, since they are present in demyelinating lesions, they are also involved in the termination of inflammation as well as producing protective factors. This is clearly seen in the cuprizone model of MS, where there is a balance of damage, regulation, and repair (22), indicating that innate immunity in MS is probably also associated both with damage and repair.

Adaptive immunity

Perivenous accumulation of T and B cells are classical pathological descriptions of active lesions in MS although such accumulations are also seen in areas of normal appearing white matter. Inflammation in the meninges and in particular B cell follicles has also been associated with cortical demyelination and grey matter damage (51, 58), although other studies have found no association (52, 57). T cells are also observed in the brain parenchyma in MS while B cells tend to be restricted to the perivascular regions. Nevertheless, the presence of B and T cells suggests that the adaptive immune system is associated with the pathology observed in MS. However, similar to microglia and macrophages discussed above, T and B cells are also regulatory, and thus the mere presence of these cells should not automatically suggest an association with the damage, but could reflect repair mechanisms.

T cells

T helper type 1 (Th1) cells secreting IFN-γ are generally considered to be the main effector T cell in MS since it is these cells that transfer EAE, the experimental animal model of MS. More recent studies indicate a more important role for Th17 CD4+ T cells. However, in contrast to CD4+ T cells, the vast majority of infiltrating lymphocytes are CD8+ T cells and these cells are more frequently associated with active lesions, and show oligoclonal expansion in the lesions. In MS T cells are associated with blood vessels. In addition to CD4+ and CD8+ T cells, $\gamma\delta$ T cells that share innate and adaptive characteristics recognise non-peptide and heat-shock proteins, for example. These cells that act as a source of innate cytokines, have been reported to make up 1–10% of T cells in MS lesions. Their role in MS is unclear, although $\gamma\delta$ T cells isolated from MS proliferate in response to HSP65 and HSP70 and induce lysis of cells that express HSP60.

In MS tissues regulatory T cells, including natural (nTreg) cells expressing the cell surface CD25 and the transcription factor forkhead box P3 (FoxP3) or inducible T regs, are observed; however, the numbers of FoxP3+ and CD4+ cells are low or undetectable (68).

B cells

As discussed above clonal expansion of B cells in MS lesions has been reported. In addition, B cell follicles have been detected in some patients (51). The role of B cells in MS is unclear, although plasmapheresis or B cell depletion with anti-CD20 antibodies is effective in MS, indicating they play a role in the pathogenesis. B cells produce cytokines that help recruit immune cells but also produce anti-inflammatory cytokines such as IL-10 and BDNF and may thus be protective and reparative. The major survival factor for B-lymphocytes, BAFF, is constitutively expressed in MS tissues, and along with CXCL12 and CXCL13 (32), which are also present in MS tissues, may aid survival and persistence of B cells in the CNS of MS patients.

Blood–brain barrier

In health the CNS is protected by the BBB, the blood–spinal cord barrier (BSCB), and the blood–CSF barrier (BCB). However, in MS these barriers are compromised, facilitating entry of leucocytes by up-regulating cell adhesion molecules. The BBB, comprised of endothelial cells, perivascular astrocytes and pericytes, is the most heavily studied of these barriers since the assumption is that MS begins with autoimmune cells migrating across a damaged BBB. The integrity of the barrier is aided by complexes called tight complexes consisting of occludin, claudins, and junctional adhesion molecules (for review see 68). The BSCB is largely similar to the BBB while the BCB barrier is comprised of epithelial cells making up the choroid plexus extensions of the ependymal lining surrounding a stroma of blood vessels that do not possess BBB properties. In addition a wide variety of agents are excluded from the CNS by a large family of efflux transporters that are located at the luminal side of the brain endothelium. Most of these transporters belong to the ATP-binding cassette protein superfamily, which actively exclude molecules from endothelia, enabling multi-drug resistance of the brain.

In MS, changes to the BBB, BSCB, and expression of MDR proteins have been reported (69), although comparative studies between the brain and spinal cord barriers in MS are lacking. As reported above, lesions in the spinal cord are more chronic than brain lesions. This could be the result of differences in the BBB and BSCB since the BSC is more permeable due to decreased levels of the multi-drug resistant protein P-glycoprotein (P-gp), as well as reduced tight junction molecules and adherence junction proteins (70).

In MS, abnormalities in junctional proteins are observed in actively demyelinating lesions as well as in normal appearing white matter (71). Surprisingly, no changes in BBB dysfunction as measured by plasma protein leakage, depositions of collagen type IV, astrogliosis, and tight junction changes are observed in grey matter lesions, indicating that BBB breakdown is not a critical event in the formation of grey matter MS lesions (47).

Conclusions

Examination of the brain and other CNS regions affected in MS is key to understanding the pathogenic mechanisms operating in the disease. Comparison with other demyelinating disease of known or suspected origin may uncover similar events in MS. In recent years the idea that autoimmunity is the cause of MS has been met with some reservation. Pathological studies have revealed an important and major contribution of neurodegeneration giving rise to the hypothesis that MS may be classified as a neurodegenerative disease. Both hypotheses have merit and ongoing research is crucial to resolve the issue. While many studies are limited to tissues from patients with long disease duration, biopsy material is available from cases very early in the disease. The lesions continually develop and regress throughout the course of the disease thus allowing the study of events in early lesion genesis, even in late stage disease. Examining the so-called pre-active lesions, thought to be the very first step in lesion formation, may reveal novel pathways operating in the disease. Continued studies using classical pathology combined with more sophisticated approaches such as microarrays and biochemical approaches will be critical to determining the cause and thus cure for MS.

Conflict of interest

Authors declare no conflict of interests.

Acknowledgements

We thank B. van der Star for helpful comments. Several of our own studies on the topic have been financially supported by the Netherlands Foundation for MS Research and the Multiple Sclerosis Society of Great Britain and Northern Ireland.

References

1. Thompson, A.J., Kermode, A.G., MacManus, D.G., *et al.* (1990). Patterns of disease activity in multiple sclerosis: clinical and magnetic resonance imaging study. *BMJ* **300**, 631–634.

2. Barkhof, F., Scheltens, P., Frequin, S.T., *et al.* (1992). Relapsing-remitting multiple sclerosis: sequential enhanced MR imaging vs clinical findings in determining disease activity. *Am. J. Roentgenol.* **159**, 1041–1047.

3. De Groot, C.J.A., Bergers, E., Kamphorst, W., *et al.* (2001). Post-mortem MRI-guided sampling of multiple sclerosis brain lesions: increased yield of actively demyelinating and (p)reactive lesions. *Brain* **124**, 1635–1645.

4. Frischer, J.M., Bramow, S., Dal-Bianco, A., *et al.* (2009). The relation between inflammation and neurodegeneration in multiple sclerosis brains. *Brain* **132**, 1175–1189.

5. Van der Valk, P. and De Groot, C.J. (2000). Staging of multiple sclerosis (MS) lesions: pathology of the time frame of MS. *Neuropathol. Appl. Neurobiol.* **26**, 2–10.

6. Geurts, J.J. and Barkhof, F. (2008). Grey matter pathology in multiple sclerosis. *Lancet Neurol.* 7, 841–851.

7. Bitsch, A., Wegener, C., da Costa, C., *et al.* (1999). Lesion development in Marburg's type of acute multiple sclerosis: from inflammation to demyelination. *Mult. Scler.* **5**, 138–146

8. Weinshenker, B.G., Wingerchuk, D.M., Pittock, S.J., Lucchinetti, C.F., and

9. Poser, C.M., Goutières, F., Carpentier, M.A., and Aicardi, J. (1986) Schilder's myelinoclastic diffuse sclerosis. *Pediatrics* **77**, 107–112.

10. Afifi, A.K., Follett, K.A., Greenlee, J., Scott, W.E., and Moore, S.A. (2001). Optic neuritis: a novel presentation of Schilder's disease. *J. Child Neurol.* **16**, 693–696.

11. Kepes, J.J. (1993). Large focal tumor-like demyelinating lesions of the brain: intermediate entity between multiple sclerosis and acute disseminated encephalomyelitis? A study of 31 patients. *Ann. Neurol.* **33**, 18–27

12. Dagher, A.P. and Smirniotopoulos, J. (1996). Tumefactive demyelinating lesions. *Neuroradiology* **38**, 560–565.

13. Wender, M. (2011). Acute disseminated encephalomyelitis (ADEM). *J. Neuroimmunol.* **231**, 92–99.

14. Dawson, J.D. (1916). The histology of disseminated sclerosis. *Trans. Royal Soc. Edin.* **50**, 517–740.

15. Green, A.J., McQuaid, S., Hauser, S.L., Allen, I.V., and Lyness, R. (2010). Ocular pathology in multiple sclerosis: retinal atrophy and inflammation irrespective of disease duration. *Brain* **133**, 1591–1601.

16. Lucchinetti, C., Brück, W., Parisi, J., *et al.* (2000). Heterogeneity of multiple sclerosis lesions: implications for the pathogenesis of demyelination. *Ann. Neurol.* **47**, 707–717.

Lennon, V.A. (2006). NMO-IgG: a specific biomarker for neuromyelitis optica. *Dis. Markers* **22**, 197–206.

17. Breij, E.C., Brink, B.P., Veerhuis, R., *et al.*
(2008). Homogeneity of active
demyelinating lesions in established
multiple sclerosis. *Ann. Neurol.* **63**, 16–25.

18. van der Goes, A., Boorsma, W., Hoekstra, K.,
et al. (2005). Determination of the sequential
degradation of myelin proteins by
macrophages. *J. Neuroimmunol.* **161**, 12–20.

19. Moore, G.R., Laule, C., Mackay, A., *et al.*
(2008). Dirty-appearing white matter in
multiple sclerosis: preliminary observations
of myelin phospholipid and axonal loss.
J. Neurol. **255**, 1802–1811.

20. Goldschmidt, T., Antel, J., König, F.B.,
Brück, W., and Kuhlmann, T. (2009).
Remyelination capacity of the MS brain
decreases with disease chronicity.
Neurology **72**, 1914–1921.

21. Albert, M., Antel, J., Brück, W., and
Stadelmann, C. (2007). Extensive cortical
remyelination in patients with chronic
multiple sclerosis. *Brain Pathol.* **17**, 129–138

22. Olah, M., Amor, S., Brouwer, N., *et al.*
(2012). Identification of a microglia
phenotype supportive of remyelination.
Glia **60**, 306–321.

23. Kipp, M., Gingele, S., Pott, F., *et al.* (2011).
BLBP-expression in astrocytes during
experimental demyelination and in human
multiple sclerosis lesions. *Brain Behav.
Immun.* **25**, 1554–1568.

24. Huizinga, R., van der Star, B.J., Kipp, M.,
et al. (2012). Phagocytosis of neuronal debris
by microglia is associated with neuronal
damage in multiple sclerosis. *Glia*, in press.

25. Dziedzic, T., Metz, I., Dallenga, T., *et al.*
(2010). Wallerian degeneration: a major
component of early axonal pathology in
multiple sclerosis. *Brain Pathol.* **20**, 976–985.

26. Wolswijk G. (2000). Oligodendrocyte
survival, loss and birth in lesions of
chronic-stage multiple sclerosis. *Brain* **123**,
105–115.

27. Barnett, M.H. and Prineas, J.W. (2004).
Relapsing and remitting multiple sclerosis:
pathology of the newly forming lesion.
Ann. Neurol. **55**, 458–468.

28. van Noort, J.M., Bsibsi, M., Gerritsen,
W.H., *et al.* (2010). Alpha B-crystallin is a
target for adaptive immune responses, and a
trigger of innate responses in preactive
multiple sclerosis lesions. *J. Neuropathol.
Exp. Neurol.* **69**, 694–703.

29. Cossins, J.A., Clements, J.M., Ford, J., *et al.*
(1997). Enhanced expression of MMP-7 and
MMP-9 in demyelinating multiple sclerosis
lesions. *Acta Neuropathol.* **94**, 590–598.

30. Raine, C.S., Bonetti, B., and Cannella, B.
(1998). Multiple sclerosis: expression of
molecules of the tumor necrosis factor
ligand and receptor families in relationship
to the demyelinated plaque. *Rev. Neurol.
(Paris)* **154**, 577–585.

31. De Groot, C.J., Ruuls, S.R., Theeuwes, J.W.,
Dijkstra, C.D., and Van der Valk, P. (1997).
Immunocytochemical characterization of
the expression of inducible and constitutive
isoforms of nitric oxide synthase in
demyelinating multiple sclerosis lesions.
J. Neuropathol. Exp. Neurol. **56**, 10–20.

32. Krumbholz, M., Theil, D., Cepok, S., *et al.*
(2006). Chemokines in multiple sclerosis:
CXCL12 and CXCL13 up-regulation is
differentially linked to CNS immune cell
recruitment. *Brain* **129**, 200–211.

33. Williams, A., Piaton, G., and Lubetzki, C.
(2007). Astrocytes – friends or foes in
multiple sclerosis? *Glia* **55**, 1300–1312.

34. Stankoff, B., Aigrot, M.S., Noël, F., *et al.*
(2002). Ciliary neurotrophic factor (CNTF)
enhances myelin formation: a novel role for
CNTF and CNTF-related molecules.
J. Neurosci. **22**, 9221–9227.

35. Harris, R.A. and Amor, S. (2011). Sweet
and sour: oxidative and carbonyl stress in
neurological disorders. *CNS Neurol. Disord.
Drug. Targets* **10**, 82–107.

36. Haider, L., Fischer, M.T., Frischer, J.M.,
et al. (2011). Oxidative damage in multiple
sclerosis lesions. *Brain* **134**, 1914–1924.

37. Nikić, I., Merkler, D., Sorbara, C., J.M.,
et al. (2011). A reversible form of axon
damage in experimental autoimmune
encephalomyelitis and multiple sclerosis.
Nat. Med. **17**, 495–499.

38. Van Noort, J.M., van Sechel, A.C.,
Bajramovic, J.J., *et al.* (1995). The small
heat shock protein alpha B-crystallin as

candidate autoantigen in multiple sclerosis. *Nature* **375**, 798–801.

39. Aquino, D.A., Capello, E., Weisstein, J., *et al.* (1997). Multiple sclerosis: altered expression of 70- and 27-kDa heat shock proteins in lesions and myelin. *J. Neuropathol. Exp. Neurol.* **56**, 664–672.

40. Stahnke, T., Stadelmann, C., Netzler, A., Brück, W., and Richter-Landsberg, C. (2007). Differential upregulation of heme oxygenase-1 (HSP32) in glial cells after oxidative stress and in demyelinating disorders. *J. Mol. Neurosci.* **32**, 25–37.

41. Gáti, I. and Leel-Ossy, L. (2001). Heat shock protein 60 in corpora amylacea. *Pathol. Oncol. Res.* **7**, 140–144.

42. Raine, C.S. (1994). Multiple sclerosis: immune system molecule expression in the central nervous system. *J. Neuropathol. Exp. Neurol.* **53**, 328–337.

43. Selmaj, K., Brosnan, C.F., and Raine, C.S. (1992). Expression of heat shock protein-65 by oligodendrocytes in vivo and in vitro: implications for multiple sclerosis. *Neurology* **42**, 795–800.

44. Stadelmann, C., Ludwin, S., Tabira, T., *et al.* (2005). Tissue preconditioning may explain concentric lesions in Balo's type of multiple sclerosis. *Brain* **128**, 979–987.

45. Van der Valk, P. and Amor, S. (2009). Preactive lesions in multiple sclerosis. *Curr. Opin. Neurol.* **22**, 207–213.

46. van Noort, J.M., van den Elsen, P.J., van Horssen, J., *et al.* (2011). Preactive multiple sclerosis lesions offer novel clues for neuroprotective therapeutic strategies. *CNS Neurol. Disord. Drug Targets* **10**, 68–81.

47. van Horssen, J., Brink, B.P., de Vries, H.E., van der Valk, P., and Bo, L. (2007). The blood-brain barrier in cortical multiple sclerosis lesions. *J. Neuropathol. Exp. Neurol.* **66**, 321–328.

48. Allen, I.V. and McKeown, S.R. (1979). A histological, histochemical, and biochemical study of the macroscopically normal white matter in multiple sclerosis. *J. Neurol. Sci.* **41**, 81–91.

49. Allen, I.V., Glover, G., and Anderson, R. (1981). Abnormalities in the macroscopically normal white matter in cases of mild or spinal multiple sclerosis. *Acta Neuropathol.* **Suppl** 7, 176–178.

50. Dutta, R. and Trapp, B.D. (2007). Pathogenesis of axonal and neuronal damage in multiple sclerosis. *Neurology* **68**, S22–31.

51. Serafini, B., Rosicarelli, B., Magliozzi, R., Stille, W., and Aloisi, F. (2004). Detection of ectopic B-cell follicles with germinal centers in the meninges of patients with secondary progressive multiple sclerosis. *Brain Pathol.* **14**, 164–174.

52. Peferoen, L.A. Lamers, F., Lodder, L.N., *et al.* (2010). Epstein Barr virus is not a characteristic feature in the central nervous system in established multiple sclerosis. *Brain* **133**, e137.

53. Lassmann, H., Niedobitek, G., Aloisi, F., and Middeldorp, J.M; NeuroProMiSe EBV Working Group. (2011). Epstein-Barr virus in the multiple sclerosis brain: a controversial issue – report on a focused workshop held in the Centre for Brain Research of the Medical University of Vienna, Austria. *Brain* **134**, 2772–2786.

54. Zeis, T., Probst, A., Steck, A.J., *et al.* (2009). Molecular changes in white matter adjacent to an active demyelinating lesion in early multiple sclerosis. *Brain Pathol.* **19**, 459–466.

55. Geurts, J.J., Stys, P.K., Minagar, A., Amor, S., and Zivadinov, R. (2009). Gray matter pathology in (chronic) MS: modern views on an early observation. *J. Neurol. Sci.* **282**, 12–20.

56. Gilmore, C.P., DeLuca, G.C., Bö, L., et al. (2009). Spinal cord neuronal pathology in multiple sclerosis. *Brain Pathol.* **19**, 642–649.

57. Kooi, E.J., Geurts, J.J., van Horssen, J., Bø, L., and van der Valk, P. (2009). Meningeal inflammation is not associated with cortical demyelination in chronic multiple sclerosis. *J. Neuropathol. Exp. Neurol.* **68**, 1021–1028.

58. Howell, O.W., Reeves, C.A., Nicholas, R., *et al.* (2011). Meningeal inflammation is widespread and linked to cortical pathology in multiple sclerosis. *Brain* **134**, 2755–2771.

59. Frischer, J.M., Bramow, S., Dal-Bianco, A., et al. (2009). The relation between inflammation and neurodegeneration in multiple sclerosis brains. *Brain* **132**, 1175–1189.

60. Bsibsi, M., Ravid, R., Gveric, D., and van Noort, J.M. (2002). Broad expression of Toll-like receptors in the human central nervous system. *J. Neuropathol. Exp. Neurol.* **61**, 1013–1021

61. Amor, S., Puentes, F., Baker, D., and van der Valk, P. (2010). Inflammation in neurodegenerative diseases. *Immunology* **129**, 154–169.

62. Ming, X., Li, W., Maeda, Y., et al. (2002). Caspase-1 expression in multiple sclerosis plaques and cultured glial cells. *Neurol. Sci.* **197**, 9–18

63. Marik, C., Felts, P.A., Bauer, J., Lassmann, H., and Smith, K.J. (2007). Lesion genesis in a subset of patients with multiple sclerosis: a role for innate immunity? *Brain* **130**, 2800–2815.

64. Lumsden, C.E. (1971). The immunogenesis of the multiple sclerosis plaque. *Brain Res.* **28**, 365–390.

65. Gay, F.W., Drye, T.J., Dick, G.W.A., and Esiri, M.M. (1997). The application of multifactorial cluster analysis in the staging of plaques in early multiple sclerosis: identification and characterization of the primary demyelinating lesion. *Brain* **120**, 1461–1483.

66. Gay, F.W. (2006). Early cellular events in multiple sclerosis: intimations of an extrinsic myelinolytic antigen. *Clin. Neurol. Neurosurg.* **108**, 234–240.

67. Zhang, Z., Zhang, Z.Y., Schittenhelm, J., et al. (2011). Parenchymal accumulation of CD163+ macrophages/microglia in multiple sclerosis brains. *J. Neuroimmunol.* **237**, 73–79.

68. Fritzsching, B., Haas, J., König, F., et al. (2011). Intracerebral human regulatory T cells: analysis of CD4+ CD25+ FOXP3+ T cells in brain lesions and cerebrospinal fluid of multiple sclerosis patients. *PLoS One* **6**, e17988.

69. Alvarez, J.I., Cayrol, R., and Prat, A. (2011). Disruption of central nervous system barriers in multiple sclerosis. *Biochim. Biophys. Acta* **1812**, 252–264.

70. Bartanusz, V., Jezova, D., Alajajian, B., and Digicaylioglu, M. (2011). The blood–spinal cord barrier: morphology and clinical implications. *Ann. Neurol.* **70**, 194–206.

71. Leech, S., Kirk, J., Plumb, J., and McQuaid, S. (2007). Persistent endothelial abnormalities and blood-brain barrier leak in primary and secondary progressive multiple sclerosis. *Neuropathol. Appl. Neurobiol.* **33**, 86–98.

Experimental autoimmune encephalomyelitis

Sandra Amor and David Baker

Background

In MS, autoimmune responses to myelin are widely considered to be responsible for demyelination and neurodegeneration in the CNS. This idea has led to the use of experimental autoimmune encephalomyelitis (EAE), a spectrum of neurological disorders following immunisation with CNS antigens, as a model of MS. The paradigm shift in MS from an autoimmune disease of myelin to that of a neurodegenerative disease has stimulated development of models in which neurodegeneration, as well as inflammation and demyelination, are observed. Thus, secondary progressive EAE, models of cortical demyelination, and experimental inflammatory neurodegenerative and spastic diseases have been developed.

In this chapter we discuss the development of EAE and review the clinical, immunological, and pathological aspects of different models. We discuss how EAE studies have been used to test therapeutic approaches and how these have translated to MS. Finally, to interpret the findings better, we address how data from EAE studies can be improved, and how this should be reported to aid better translation to MS.

History of EAE

In 1880, rabies infection of humans was relatively common. To investigate his 'germ hypothesis' Louis Pasteur developed vaccinations for several diseases, including rabies, by preparing freeze-dried spinal cord tissue from rabies-infected rabbits. In 1885 Pasteur injected a 9-year-old boy who had been bitten by a rabid dog with a series of immunisations. When batches of the vaccine proved less effective in a larger group of subjects, Pasteur increased the frequency of injections using more potent vaccines prepared from rapid freeze-drying procedures. As a result, sporadic reports of vaccine-associated paralysis were reported that, in the most severe forms, were fatal (1). These side effects were not related to rabies virus infection itself since hydrocephalous, a typical clinical sign of rabies infections, and rabies-induced neuronal death were not observed. Rather, the pathology revealed extensive inflammation and perivenous demyelination in the brain and spinal cord more typical of an allergic reaction. It was these early studies that stimulated virologist Thomas Rivers' interest in neurological complications following viral infections and vaccinations. In the 1930s Rivers reproduced Pasteur's findings in rhesus monkeys and rabbits

The Biology of Multiple Sclerosis, ed Gregory J. Atkins, Sandra Amor, Jean M. Fletcher and Kingston H.G. Mills. Published by Cambridge University Press. © Gregory J. Atkins, Sandra Amor, Jean M. Fletcher and Kingston H.G. Mills 2012.

and, surprisingly, induced paralysis in animals injected with tissues from non-infected control animals (2). Again, the pathology resembled human paralytic inflammatory demyelinating disease, verifying that the disease was not due to the rabies virus infection. Thus, associations between the immune response and the paralytic disease led to the assumption that autoimmunity to CNS antigens caused the disease. This hypothesis gave rise to the name experimental allergic encephalomyelitis or experimental autoimmune encephalomyelitis as it is more commonly known.

While Rivers' studies required many repeated injections of brain tissues, Kabat found that by augmenting the immune response using an adjuvant developed by Freund (3), the experimental disease could be induced using only a few injections, and that EAE could be induced within weeks rather than months (4). Such immunisations of rhesus monkeys induced a relapsing–remitting paralytic illness in which paralysis occurred in different limbs and animals displayed different neurological symptoms with each disease episode. The similarities between this experimentally induced encephalitis and MS, as well as post-infectious disorders, led to the hypothesis that these human diseases were also due to an allergic reaction. The myelin damage observed in the immunised animals directed attention to the identification of myelin antigens thought to provoke this 'autoimmune response'. The findings from Pasteur and followers and later key studies in the search for the autoantigen and mechanisms involved in EAE are summarised in Table 3.1 and are addressed in more detail below.

Induction of EAE

Induction of EAE relies on the generation of autoreactive T cells. This is achieved following active immunisation of the autoantigen emulsified in an adjuvant (active EAE), or by generating activated T cells in vitro and transferring the cells to naïve recipient animals (passive or adoptive transfer EAE). The disease course, severity, and pathological features observed in the CNS are dependent on the choice of autoantigen and adjuvant, as well as the species, strain, gender, and age of the animals.

Adjuvants

Since the early studies of Rivers and Kabat, adjuvants are known to augment the immunological response to autoantigens to obtain reproducible disease. The mode of action of adjuvants was originally thought to be via boosting the antibody responses. It is now known that adjuvants, which frequently contain killed mycobacterium, also elicit T cell responses via toll-like receptor (TLR) activation (5). This is explained by the fact that viruses, bacteria, and altered-self antigens trigger the innate immune response via TLR activation. Such innate immune activation is necessary for triggering the adaptive immune responses, such as the T helper 1 (Th1) responses, or Th17 responses when *Citrobacter rodentium* is used (6). In the case of EAE, the response to myelin triggers production of TNFα, important for disease induction. The first adjuvant in EAE studies was that designed by Freund, an adjuvant consisting of an oil-in-water emulsion called incomplete Freund's adjuvant (IFA). When inactivated dried mycobacteria are added to IFA this is called complete Freund's adjuvant (CFA). EAE can also be induced with IFA containing bacterial preparations of *M. butyricum* and *Bordetella pertussis* (5) (Table 3.2). For some mouse strains an additional immunological boost is required in the form of pertussis toxin derived from *B. pertussis* (7). It is still debatable how pertussis toxin augments EAE although non-selective expansion

Table 3.1 Timeline showing milestones in the history of EAE

Date	Event
1885	Louis Pasteur produces rabies vaccine and injects a boy bitten by a rabid dog
1887	Paralytic illness in humans following vaccine immunisation
1933	Repeated immunisation of macaques induces paralysis and myelin damage
1942	Freund produces adjuvant
1947	Use of adjuvant to augment responses to CNS antigens
1949	Induction of EAE in mice with mouse brain tissue
1954	Induction of EAE with white matter
1960	Adoptive transfer of EAE with T cells directed to myelin
1961	Use of anti-serum directed to lymphocytes suppresses EAE
1969	EAE induction with MBP peptides
1971	Use of glatiramer acetate to treat EAE
1981	Transfer of EAE with CD4+ T cells
1982	Identification of MBP epitope 89–169 in SJL mice
1987	Antibodies to MOG augment EAE disease
1985	Induction of EAE in guinea pigs with PLP
1987	Use of mitoxantrone to suppress EAE
1988	Inhibition of EAE following oral tolerance with MBP
1989	Use of altered peptide ligands of MBP inhibits EAE
1992	Treatment of EAE with antibodies to VLA-4
1994	EAE with recombinant MOG and MOG peptides in mice
1998	Role of regulatory CD4+ CD25+ cells
2000	Reduction of EAE in complement-deficient mice
2001	Transfer of EAE with CD8+ cells
2003	Use of stem cells
2003	EAE in humanised DR2 transgenic mouse
2004	Induction of optic neuritis in rhesus macaques with OSP
2005	Therapy blocking IL-17
2007	Antibodies to neurofascin augment neuronal damage in rats
2007	Immunisation with NF-L induces neuronal damage in mice
2008	Secondary progressive EAE model defined
2011	DNA vaccinations in EAE
2011	Use of rituximab in EAE
2011	Cortical demyelination in EAE models

ABH – antibody high, IL – interleukin, NF-L – neurofilament light, MBP – myelin basic protein, MOG – myelin oligodendrocyte glycoprotein, PLP – proteolipid protein, OSP – oligodendrocyte-specific protein.

Table 3.2 Adjuvants used in EAE

Adjuvant	Component and comment
Freund's incomplete (IFA)	Oil-in-water (3,11)
Freund's complete (CFA)	Killed mycobacterium of *Mycobacterium tuberculosis; M. butyricum, Bordetella pertussis, Citrobacter rodentium* (5,6)
Alum	Provokes Th2 response (5)
B. pertussis toxin	Mechanism of action thought to be due to changes in BBB and activation of Th1 and Th17 cells (8)
DNA vaccine and CpG motifs	Modulation of the immune response (9)
Carbonyl iron	Metallic iron characterised by spherical particles (10)
Muramyl dipeptide	Water-soluble adjuvant (N-acetyl-muramyl L-alanyl D-isoglutamine; MDP) in IFA (12)

of autoreactive T cells and changes in the blood–brain barrier (BBB) have been proposed (7,8), with the former being the most likely reason for the efficacy. With the knowledge that different components activate TLR, CpG motifs have also been added to IFA to induce EAE (9). The importance of adjuvants for the induction of EAE is observed using rats. Lewis rats are considered susceptible, while Brown Norway rats are resistant. However, when Brown Norway rats are immunised with adjuvant containing carbonyl ion, rather than mycobacterium, they develop EAE (10). Thus adjuvants differentially activate the innate immune system, indicating that different routes of innate immune activation play a role in inducing disease in different models.

Other adjuvants include the aluminium salts, aluminium hydroxide, and aluminium phosphate, collectively known as Alum. These were originally used in vaccine preparations for veterinary practice but are also used in human vaccines. Alums may also be used as adjuvants for induction of EAE, but provoke a protective Th2 response. For EAE induction, several adjuvants can be used (Table 3.2) although the most widely used adjuvant is CFA. Nevertheless, some rat strains do not require addition of mycobacterium. Chronic relapsing EAE (CR-EAE) in the Dark Agouti (DA) rat can be induced with myelin proteins in IFA (11) making this model more desirable for ethical reasons since mycobacterium can cause side effects.

Autoantigens

Myelin proteins. That autoimmune responses to myelin antigens may play a role in the pathogenesis of MS inspired the search for the target antigens. Early studies took advantage of the high solubility and ease of purification of myelin basic protein (MBP). Thus MBP was used extensively to examine if autoimmune responses were present in MS patients, and whether immunisation with MBP could induce EAE (13). Other than MBP, myelin is composed of many different proteins as well as lipids. Examining human CNS myelin reveals the presence of many myelin-associated proteins. As observed in Figure 3.1A, MBP and proteolipid protein (PLP) are the dominant proteins in myelin. The major isoform of

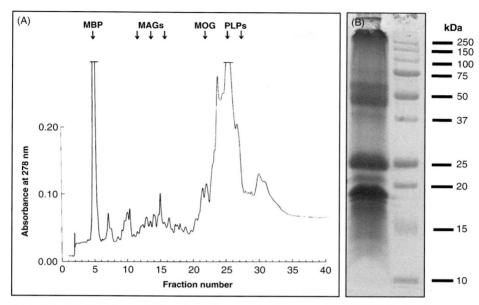

Figure 3.1. Delipidated human CNS myelin was fractionated using reverse phase-HPLC (A). The low fraction numbers indicate hydrophilic proteins such as MBP and high fraction numbers the hydrophobic proteins such as PLP. (B) SDS-PAGE gel separation of proteins in human MS myelin stained with Coomasie Blue. (Data courtesy of Dr. J.M. van Noort.)

MBP has a molecular weight of 18.5 kDa (see Figure 3.1B) and represents about 30% of the total myelin proteins. MBP is localised exclusively at the cytoplasmic surface of the major dense lines and helps stabilise the myelin sheath. The protein is composed of several isoforms, some of which are also present in peripheral myelin.

The major myelin protein is proteolipid protein (PLP), constituting about 50% of the total protein. PLP has a molecular weight of 25–30 kDa and is found only in the CNS. An isoform of PLP, DM20, is generated by alternative RNA splicing, lacking 35 residues from an intracellular loop. PLP is a transmembrane protein that is highly hydrophobic, often making EAE immunisation procedures difficult. The crucial role of PLP is shown in PLP-deficient mice that develop widespread axonal damage and degeneration, while defective PLP-expressing mice exhibit hypomyelination and early death.

For many years MBP and PLP were the only proteins used to induce EAE; however, with more sophisticated biochemical and molecular techniques it has been possible to identify and purify the minor proteins. One minor protein, myelin oligodendrocyte glycoprotein (MOG), has been the focus of many MS and EAE studies. MOG has a molecular weight of 25 kDa and makes up only 2.5% of total white matter myelin of the CNS (14). The function of MOG within the CNS is speculated to be an 'adhesion molecule' providing structural integrity to the myelin sheath. MOG has provoked interest in both MS and EAE studies since not only is the protein CNS-specific, but it is also expressed on the surface of mature oligodendrocytes and myelin, making it an ideal target of the immune response. Another protein of interest in EAE and MS is myelin-associated glycoprotein (MAG), a quantitatively minor 100 kDa glycoprotein representing 1% of the total protein. MAG belongs to the Ig superfamily and is present in both the CNS and peripheral nervous system (PNS). In the CNS, MAG is located on the inner membrane of myelin in close contact with the axon. Given its structure, it has been proposed that MAG acts as an adhesion and signaling molecule between oligodendrocytes/myelin and axons. MAG exists as L-MAG and S-MAG, depending on the (Long or Short) length of the cytoplasmic tail. Other proteins of relevance to EAE and MS are oligodendrocyte-myelin glycoprotein (OMgp) and oligodendrocyte-specific protein (OSP). OMgp is a 110 kDa glycoprotein located on myelin and oligodendrocytes, and in neurons where it is implicated in growth cone collapse and inhibition of neurite outgrowth. The tetraspanin OSP, also known as claudin-11, is found in the radial component of myelin and is important in the tight junctions. Another minor protein, 2':3'-cyclic nucleotide 3'-phosphodiesterase (CNPase), differentially expressed during ageing, appears as a doublet of 46 kDa and 48 kDa in myelin. CNPase is expressed highly in oligodendrocytes, at low levels on other cell types, and Schwann cells. The function of CNPase is thought to be in binding of cytoskeletal elements and promoting outgrowth of processes in non-neuronal cells.

Myelin-associated heat-shock proteins. Examination of MS myelin compared to control myelin has revealed the expression of the stress protein alpha B crystallin in myelin and oligodendrocytes in the CNS of people with MS including cells in pre-active MS lesions. Alpha B crystallin is the dominant antigen for T cell and antibody response in both MS patients and healthy controls (15,16). However, immunisation of the protein fails to induce EAE in many mouse strains, probably due to immune tolerance as a result of its expression in the thymus. Nevertheless, the cryptic epitope 1–16 induces mild disease in ABH mice (17) associated with the lack of expression of alpha B crystallin in these mice.

Neuronal proteins. Neurons and axons also act as targets of the immune response (18–20). The target proteins include the cytoskeleton protein neurofilament light (NF-L), a 68–70 kDa protein, that with NF-medium and NF-heavy is crucial for the function of the axons. In NF-L-deficient mice axonal transport is inhibited resulting in axonal hypotrophy and neurodegeneration. Another neuronal antigen, linked to MS and EAE, is neurofascin, present at the paranodal junctions and important for the stability of the myelin-axon unit. The two forms of neurofascin based on their molecular weights are neurofascin 186, a neuronal protein concentrated in myelinated fibres at nodes of Ranvier, and neurofascin 155, which is the oligodendrocyte-specific isoform. Mice lacking neurofascin develop a progressive deterioration of the paranodal structure. Another juxtanodal protein is contactin-2 (TAG-1), present on the axolemma, myelin sheath, and on neurons, where it is thought to be involved in clustering of axonal voltage-gated potassium channels.

Aquaporin 4. Autoimmunity to astrocytic proteins has also been implicated in demyelinating disease. In *neuromyelitis optica*, a demyelinating disease in which the damage preferentially occurs in the optic nerve and spinal cord, antibodies to the water channel aquaporin 4, present in patients, induce similar pathology in experimental animals, revealing the first autoimmune disease in the CNS.

In summary, autoimmunity to CNS myelin, neuronal antigens, and astrocytes, as well as proteins expressed during disease, induce neurological disease in animals. The mechanisms of action of the pathogenic responses and their role in EAE will be discussed in detail later in this chapter.

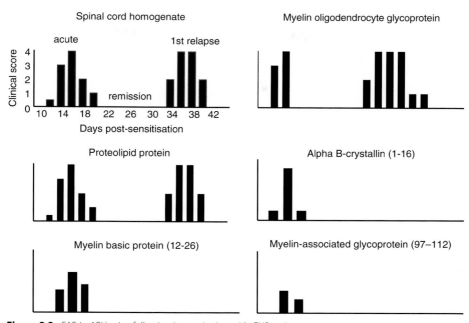

Figure 3.2. EAE in ABH mice following immunisation with CNS antigens.

Immunisation protocols

Protocols for EAE induction vary among laboratories, species, and models indicating a real need for standardisation to enable comparisons of studies. With the development of the principles of the 3Rs (Reduction, Refinement, and Replacement) EAE protocols are undergoing reassessment by researchers, journals, and ethical review boards. Protocols that lead to severe discomfort, e.g. footpad injections once commonly used to induce EAE in rats and guinea pigs, have been banned. Also some routes of injection of adjuvants, e.g. subcutaneous, are preferred since intradermal injections cause skin ulceration and necrosis and are painful. Few papers report the exact details of EAE protocols making it difficult to repeat published studies. Recently, a detailed description of EAE in ABH mice has been reported (21, 22). Brief details of this protocol using SCH-induced EAE in ABH mice is given here to explain the complexity of immunisations. This protocol has also been used for EAE induced with PLP, MOG, MBP, MAG, OSP, CNPase, alpha B-crystallin, and NF-L (18, 23) (Figure 3.2).

EAE protocol for ABH mice

Preparation of adjuvant. A stock solution of CFA is made by adding 16 mg of *M. tuberculosis* H37Ra and 2 mg of *M. butyricum* to 4 ml of IFA. This can be stored for 1 month at 4°C. To prepare the working solution 1 ml of CFA stock is added to 11.5 ml of IFA. To prepare sufficient emulsion for 25 mice, remove the plunger from a 20 ml syringe and plug the end of the barrel. To the syringe, add 5 ml of sterile phosphate buffered saline and 33 mg of freeze-dried SCH and vortex gently. Add 5 ml of the working solution of CFA and gently mix. Cover the open end (top) of the syringe with parafilm and gently vortex.

Table 3.3 Clinical signs of EAE in mice

EAE score	Neurological deficit
0	Healthy
1	Limp tail
2	Impaired righting reflex
3	Partial hind-limb paralysis
4	Complete hind-limb paralysis
5	Moribund/death

Sonicate for 10 minutes to allow the SCH to dissociate. To make the emulsion for injection use a 1 ml syringe to pump the emulsion until thick enough such that a drop of the emulsion does not disperse on water. Slowly, remove the plug and replace the syringe plunger into the barrel gently tapping the barrel to ensure the emulsion does not leak from the end. Use a long (6 cm) large bore needle (e.g. needle for taking CSF samples). Prepare 1 ml syringes for injections by withdrawing the barrel until the 1 ml mark. Insert the large bore needle into the 1 ml syringes and carefully fill them avoiding air bubbles. Remove oil from the 1 ml syringe and firmly fix on 16 mm, 25 g needles for injection.

Injection of adjuvant. Adult 8- to 10-week-old mice are immunised subcutaneously with 300 µl adjuvant using two injections of 150 µl in two spots on the back. The first of these injections is performed on day 0 and the second 1 week later. When EAE is induced using peptides, immediately and 24 hours after immunisation, the mice are injected intraperitoneally with 200 ng of pertussis toxin.

Clinical scoring

The disease course of EAE depends on the immunisation protocol, animal strain, and species. The first signs of neurological disease in acute monophasic EAE are generally observed between 10 and 17 days following immunisation. Adoptive transfer of encephalitogenic T cells induces disease somewhat earlier than active disease, i.e. 5–7 days after cell transfer. The clinical signs of disease are recorded on a scale of 0–5 (Table 3.3). In addition to the signs typical of EAE, neurological disease can be monitored using a rotor rod, extent of bladder dysfunction, as well as behavioural changes. Prior to onset of EAE, weight changes are observed and may be useful, although not consistent, to predict onset (21).

Disease courses

Immunisation of susceptible animals with CNS tissues and adjuvant, or following adoptive transfer of T cells, frequently elicits a monophasic neurological disease termed acute EAE (Figure 3.2). After the peak of disease animals recover and return to baseline, termed the remission phase. In some models animals do not recover and develop a chronic paralytic disease as seen in C57BL/6 mice immunised with MOG[35-55]. In some EAE models, animals develop CR-EAE as shown with SCH, MOG, and PLP (Figure 3.2). ABH mice immunised with SCH recover from the relapse after which they develop subsequent relapses in which neurological deficits accumulate to progressive disability – so-called secondary progressive EAE (24) (Table 3.4).

Table 3.4 Spectrum of EAE

Species	EAE	Model	Reference
Mouse	Acute monophasic	ABH. Active immunisation with MBP, MAG, alpha B-crystallin	17, 25, 26
	Chronic	C57BL/6, ABH. Active immunisation with MOG[35–55]	23
	Secondary progressive	ABH. Immunisation with SCH in CFA	22, 24
	Spastic paresis	ABH. Active immunisation with NF-L	18, 27
	CR-EAE	ABH. Active immunisation with rMOG, MOG[8–21], PLP, PLP[56–70], SCH	22, 28, 29
Rat	Hyperacute	Lewis. Adoptive transfer of MBP T cells	30
	Acute monophasic	Lewis. Active immunisation with MBP, MOG, PLP or adoptive transfer with MOG, MBP, GFAP, S-100B	31
	CR-EAE	DA. Immunisation with rMOG, SCH in IFA	11
Guinea pig	Acute	Hartley. Immunisation with myelin, MBP	12, 32, 33
	Acute, CR-EAE	Juvenile strain 13. Immunisation with SCH in CFA	
	Chronic progressive		
Marmoset	Acute	High doses of mycobacteria in CFA plus *Bordetella pertussis* is necessary	34
	Chronic	rMOG in CFA, MOG-in-myelin in CFA	35
Rhesus macaque	Acute	High doses of myelin in CFA lead to fast progressive disease	36
	CR-EAE	Homologous MBP in CFA. Inflammation and demyelination	37
	Acute with optic neuritis	OSP in CFA	38

Choice of model
Mice

Although many animals are susceptible to EAE (Table 3.4), mice are the most common rodents used since many biological tools and transgenic animals are available to probe the disease. Initially only acute EAE in the mouse was available, but by adaptation of the protocol and changing the antigen, mice developed CR-EAE by active sensitisation or adoptive T cell transfer (39, 40). In the adoptive transfer EAE models, animals are immunised with CNS antigens and the spleen and lymph nodes collected at day 10. Single cell suspensions are cultured for 3 days with the antigen and transferred into naïve recipient animals. Disease is observed between 5 and 10 days after cell transfer.

EAE was largely restricted to MBP for immunisation in SJL (H-2^s) and PL/J (H-2^u) mice. While the more hydrophobic PLP is difficult to use, the protein and peptides induce EAE in SJL and ABH mice (28, 41) (Table 3.5). In an attempt to model the clinical course and pathology of MS better, the CNS-specific protein MOG was used, since antibodies to MOG are pathogenic in mice. The recombinant protein, peptides and

Table 3.5 Encephalitogenic peptides in mice and rats

	MHC class II	MBP	PLP	MOG
Mouse				
ABH	g7	1–12	56–70	8–21, 35–55, 43–57
SJL	s	17–27, 89–101	139–151, 178–191	92–106
PLJ	u	Ac1–9, 33–35	43–64	35–55
C57BL/6	b	nd	nd	35–55
Rat				
Lewis	1	68–86, 87–99	nd	1–20, 91–108, 103–125
Dark Agouti	av1	63–81, 101–120, 142–167	nd	74–90, 93–107
Brown Norway	n	nd	nd	21–38

nd – not determined.

native MOG-in-myelin, are encephalitogenic in SJL and ABH (H-2^{dq1}) mice (14, 29), as well as C57BL/6 (H-2^b) on which many genetically modified mice are generated. A disadvantage of EAE in C57BL/6 mice is the chronicity of disease (42), preventing study of mechanisms involved in relapse and remissions. In mouse models, age, gender, and environmental factors influence EAE susceptibility. For example, in SJL mice immunised with PLP, young male mice are relatively resistant whereas older males and SJL females are susceptible. Intriguingly, older mice immunised in winter are more susceptible to EAE (43) indicating an effect of environmental factors on disease suscepti-bility as observed in MS.

Rats

Lewis, Brown Norway, Dark Agouti (DA), and Wistar strains are commonly used. Rats offer advantages of size, requirements for very low doses of antigen, and pertussis toxin is not required. EAE in the Lewis rat is an acute paralytic disease in which demyelination is uncommon. In contrast, CR-EAE occurs in DA rats immunised with MOG or SCH emulsified in IFA. The size of the animals offers an advantage for fine manipulations, such as induction of discrete focal lesions in the spinal cord useful for transplanting stem cells. Gender and age influence EAE susceptibility in Wistar rats since young animals develop acute EAE and remission, whereas middle-aged males develop severe chronic EAE (44).

Guinea pigs

In the 1960s Hartley and juvenile strain 13 guinea pigs were widely used for EAE studies. Protocols included sensitisation with myelin or MBP in CFA, in which MDP could replace mycobacterium (12). CR-EAE was observed in the strain 13 guinea pigs immunised with whole CNS homogenates, and became the model of choice at the time. Pathologically, the large lesions observed in the strain 13 guinea pigs immunised with whole CNS homogenates better resemble MS than any other model. PLP has also been reported to induce demyelinating EAE in Hartley guinea pigs while strain 13 guinea pigs are resistant (45). While these models appear superior to murine models due to the lack of appropriate tools, e.g. monoclonal antibodies to probe the disease, guinea pigs are less popular than previously.

Marmosets

Common marmosets (*Callithrix jacchus*) give birth to young that in utero share placental blood circulation. This allows adoptive transfer EAE as well as using twin pairs for comparative EAE studies, which is not possible in other out-bred animals. Following immunisation with human myelin in CFA, marmosets develop a relapsing–remitting disease course in which demyelination is observed (34). The model has since been refined using recombinant MOG and reducing the mycobacteria, showing demyelination, inflammation, and axonal pathology (46) in the CNS that is amenable to MRI to monitor disease.

Rhesus macaques

The evolutionary distance between rhesus monkeys and humans is estimated at 35 million years. The rhesus macaque (*Macaca mulatta*) was the first animal shown to be susceptible to EAE (2) and develops disease following immunisation with SCH, human myelin, human MBP, and recombinant human MOG in CFA. All develop a severe hyperacute clinical disease that progresses rapidly to death within 12 to 24 hours (36, 37, 47). This acute EAE resembles Marburg's disease. Also optic neuritis and blindness, symptoms of MS, are observed in rhesus monkeys immunised with OSP (38).

Pathology of EAE
Localisation of lesions

EAE lesions in rodents are largely restricted to the spinal cord and optic nerve (Figure 3.3), although brain lesions are observed in the cerebellum in later stages of EAE and chronic disease, but do not correlate with clinical neurological disease. In non-human primates, lesions are observed throughout the CNS. Why lesions are localised in some EAE models is unclear. Transgenic mice, in which genes for cytokines and chemokines are differentially expressed in the CNS, reveal that recruitment of pathogenic cells may depend on local expression of recruitment factors. Also, differential expression of the target autoantigen may control autoreactive T cell recruitment. Pathogenic cells are generally excluded from the CNS by the BBB or blood–spinal cord barrier (BSCB). The functional and morphological differences between the BBB and BSCB may control influx into different regions of the CNS (48). Finally, different populations of oligodendrocytes (the target of autoimmunity) colonise the spinal cord and different brain regions. Whether the ancestry of the oligodendrocytes influences susceptibility to autoimmunity, apoptosis, and death pathways is unknown. In summary, several factors may dictate regional differences of lesions in EAE. This remains to be clarified, yet could be an important clue as to why the lesions arise in EAE as well as in MS.

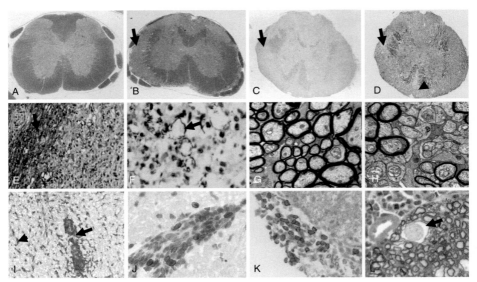

Figure 3.3. Pathology of EAE in mice. Spinal cord section of control Biozzi mice showing normal myelin (A) compared to loss of myelin (arrows) in relapse EAE. (B) toludine blue stain and (C) luxol fast blue stain. Demyelination is directly associated with axonal loss (D) as shown using Bielshowsky silver impregnation technique in which remaining axons are black (arrowhead). In more detail normal myelin (arrow E) compared to only remnants of myelin in mice with acute EAE co-injected with a monoclonal antibody to MOG (F). Similarly, electronmicroscopical studies of normal myelin (G) and naked axons in EAE (H). Inflammation in acute EAE showing activation of macrophages in the perivascular space (I, arrow) and activated microglia (I, arrowhead), CD3 positive T cells (J) and B cells (K). Axonal degeneration in Biozzi mice following immunisation with NF-L shows swollen axons (L arrow). See plate section for colour version.

Demyelination

Myelin damage, as observed in MS, can be either a primary or secondary feature (see Figure 3.3). Primary demyelination is observed in the so-called 'outside-in' model (49) in which inflammatory demyelination leads to secondary axonal swelling and degeneration. Pathologically this is observed as naked axons. Alternatively, in the 'inside-out' model, selective degeneration of axons (wallerian degeneration) is followed by demyelination only as a secondary step. In the latter situation, the presence of empty 'myelin sheaths' is probably the result of myelin debris following degeneration of axons. Whether either situation arises from a local insult, such as activated microglia, antibodies, or T cells, or is the result of axonal degeneration from an 'upstream' lesion is unknown. It is highly likely that both outside-in and inside-out pathogenic mechanisms play a role in the demyelination observed in EAE.

Rodent models rarely show primary myelin damage in the acute phase; thus primary demyelination is best studied in chronic relapsing models, or models in which animals are immunised with recombinant MOG, since antibodies to MOG are associated with myelin damage. The best model for studying demyelination is CR-EAE in the strain 13 guinea pig immunised with whole CNS tissue. Demyelination is also characteristic of MOG-induced EAE in rats and marmosets. While the advantage of the larger animals is the possibility to use imaging techniques, the manipulations are expensive and difficult to control statistically, due to the low numbers available.

Despite early descriptions of cortical demyelination in MS, little attention has been paid to this in existing EAE models. However, myelin damage is present in the cortex of mice and marmosets with EAE (46, 50), indicating that some models may reflect the cortical damage in MS.

Remyelination

Recovery from clinical disease is associated with remyelination and repair in EAE as observed in mice, rats, and guinea pigs. One feature of remyelination is the presence and division of endogenous oligodendrocyte precursor cells (OPCs) (identified by NG-2 expression) and differentiation into mature oligodendrocytes. OPCs are observed following relapses in CR-EAE in rats and mice and are observed in both the white and grey matter. In chronic MOG^{35-55} -EAE in C57BL/6 mice, the numbers of OPCs diminish or fail to develop into mature oligodendrocytes (50), although whether this is the cause or effect of chronic disease is unknown. As well as mobilizing local OPCs, Schwann cells may also populate the CNS, aiding remyelination particularly in regions close to nerve root entry zones.

Oligodendrocyte damage and death

Oligodendrocyte death in EAE is more frequently observed in CR-EAE models and MOG-induced EAE. The use of EAE in transgenic mice reveals several pathways involved in oligodendrocyte damage and death. For example, due to their high metabolic rates and energy consumption oligodendrocytes are very susceptible to oxidative damage. These cells also have high stores of iron as a requirement in myelin production pathways, which render the cells susceptible to free radical damage and lipid peroxidation (52). Conversely, the relatively low levels of antioxidants may contribute to such damage. Oligodendrocytes also express receptors for glutamate, further increasing susceptibility to exocytotoxicity.

Autoimmune mechanisms of cell death include direct attack by myelin-reactive T cells or antibody-mediated damage via complement pathways. In the latter case antibodies to MOG augment demyelination in acute EAE (50), damage cells in vitro, and may induce stress responses, making oligodendrocytes susceptible to bystander mechanisms. Yet further, as in NMO, damage to astrocytes may subsequently lead to oligodendrocyte death (53). Inflammatory mediators present in EAE lesions include TNFα. TNFα may induce apoptosis of oligodendrocytes via a number of pathways. Members of the TNF family, and TNF-Receptor superfamily, are important in mediating apoptosis via ligand interaction such as Fas-FasL, TRAIL/TRAIL receptor, and TNFα/TNF-R1. Transgenic and knock-out mice reveal an important role for Fas-FasL interactions as well as TNF-R1-induced apoptosis of oligodendrocytes. This is supported by the finding that transgenic mice, deficient in both Fas in oligodendrocyte and TNF-R1, are almost resistant to EAE (54). Also a role for the death receptor 6 (DR6), an orphan member of the TNF-R superfamily, is suggested by the finding that over-expression of DR6 in oligodendrocytes leads to caspase-3 activation and cell death, while treatment with an antagonist antibody promotes remyelination in EAE (55).

Neurodegeneration and axonal damage

That cortical demyelination, axonal damage, and neurodegeneration are present in the CNS in MS lesions, stimulated the development of EAE models to also reflect these aspects.

Axonal damage is present in EAE since neurofilament is present in the CSF of affected animals. In addition, cortical deep grey matter demyelination is present in some EAE models (46, 56). Similar to myelin, autoimmunity to axons and neurons also contributes to disease as shown in some models. For example, immunisation with NF-L, tau or passive transfer of antibodies to neurofascin and contact-2 induce and augment neuronal damage and axonal degeneration in experimental animals (18, 20, 28, 57, 58). In NF-L-immunised mice axonal damage is a direct result of responses of autoimmunity to the cytoskeletal protein as observed by the presence of empty myelin sheaths in areas where the myelin is still intact (Figure 3.3). Moreover, immunoglobulin is deposited on axonal structures in contrast to MOG-immunised animals where immunoglobulin is deposited on myelin. In CR-EAE models extensive axonal damage is also observed in the secondary progressive phase in ABH mice immunised with whole spinal cord homogenate (22, 24), reflecting the pathological picture in MS.

Astrocyte pathology

Astrogliosis as a result of hyperplasia and hypertrophy of astrocytes leads to glial scars identified by strong expression of glial fibrillary acid protein (GFAP). Gliotic scars are reported in many EAE models, especially guinea pig models and chronic EAE in ABH mice (24). Why astrocytes become hypertrophic is unclear, although accumulation of carbonylated GFAP in chronic EAE has been suggested to underlie the exaggerated morphology of astrocytes in mice. Conversely, EAE studies in mice show diminished GFAP and aquaporin 4 in early disease, suggesting damage to astrocytes during disease. Astrocytes are a critical component of the BBB and thus astrocyte pathology may contribute to BBB disturbances in EAE. Blocking astrogliosis in a conditional transgenic mouse exacerbated established EAE due to increased macrophage infiltration and associated proinflammatory response (59). Astrocytes also have a protective role in EAE by regulating macrophages, suppressing pathogenic Th17 cells, and induction of regulatory T cells.

BBB and vascular damage

As well as the BBB and the BSCB the CNS is also protected by the blood–cerebrospinal fluid barrier (BCB) of the choroid plexus. In EAE barrier damage is thought to facilitate leucocyte infiltration and thus disease. Although the precise mechanisms involved in barrier breakdown are unclear, several potentially disruptive mediators have been implicated including selectins, chemokines, integrins, and matrix metalloproteinases, which allow the migration of leucocytes across the BBB and into the CNS parenchyma. Restoring integrity of the barriers is a major aim of drug therapies.

The extent of barrier leakage can be imaged using MRI or with small ion particles. These have revealed that macrophages cross an intact BBB while pathogenic antibodies require a leaky barrier. Immunocytochemistry shows increased expression of cell adhesion molecules during clinical disease that decreases in remission. Further support is seen by leakage of pathogenic antibodies (50). Another sign of BBB disturbance is the reduction in expression of the multi-drug resistance protein p-glycoprotein in regions of perivascular inflammation. Whether this can be used to the advantage of targeting drugs to lesions is under investigation.

Table 3.6 Innate immunity in EAE

Component	Model	Expression or impact on EAE
TLR4	C57BL/6 TLR4 null mice. MOG$^{35-55}$	More severe EAE
TLR9	C57BL/6 TLR9 null mice. MOG$^{35-55}$	More severe EAE and pathology
AGE/RAGE	B10.PL mice. MBP^{ac1-9}	Blocking RAGE suppresses EAE
Adenosine receptors	C57BL/6 A1AR null mice. MOG$^{35-55}$	Severe progressive EAE
Complement	Lewis rats or ABH mice. Antibody augmented EAE	Cobra venom factor reduces clinical signs. C5 protects and promotes remyelination
Macrophages and microglia	C57BL/6 MOG$^{35-55}$ or Lewis rat MBP. Clodronate blockage	Reduced EAE when treated prior to induction but ineffective when used after induction
Mast cells	Mast cell deficient C57BL/6 W(-sh). MOG$^{35-55}$ SJL-Kit(W/W-v). PLP$^{139-151}$	More severe acute EAE Reduced EAE yet relapses intact
γδ T cells	Depletion	Reduced EAE
NK cells	C57BL/6. MOG$^{35-55}$	Regulation and inhibition of EAE

Immune mechanisms
Innate immunity

Although EAE is considered to be a CD4+ T cell-mediated disease, activation of the innate immune response is critical for disease induction. Omission of mycobacterium in the adjuvant, in general, does not lead to clinical disease, since activation of the innate immune system is required for activation of the adaptive immune response. The innate immune system encompasses phagocytic cells (e.g. monocytes and macrophages), cells that release inflammatory mediators (e.g. mast cells), natural killer (NK) cells, and molecules such as complement proteins and acute phase proteins.

Pathogen/pattern recognition receptors. Innate immune cells recognise evolutionarily conserved structures via pattern recognition receptors (PRRs). These include toll-like receptors (TLRs), nucleotide-oligomerization domain leucine-rich repeat (NOD-LRR) proteins, and cytoplasmic caspase activation and recruiting domain helicases such as retinoic-acid-inducible gene I (RIG-I)-like helicases (RLHs). These receptors are key to initiating the innate immune response and regulate the adaptive immune response to infection or tissue injury. Table 3.6 shows examples of aspects of the innate immune system's impact on either development, or severity, of EAE (60, 61).

Macrophages and microglia in EAE are critical for disease and are the dominant cell type in lesions. In EAE these cells upregulate MHC class II, co-stimulatory molecules, TLRs, adhesion molecules, and secrete cytokines and chemokines allowing recruitment of adaptive immune cells and antigen presentation. In addition, macrophages and microglia produce free radicals, matrix metalloproteinase, and glutamate, which contribute to myelin damage and neurodegeneration. The plasticity of macrophages/microglia is reflected by the ability to control disease by expression of anti-inflammatory molecules. In EAE lesions macrophages phagocytose myelin and allow removal of cell debris, critical for effective repair.

Complement. Cobra venom factor effectively reduces signs of antibody-augmented EAE, indicating a role for complement in disease. More detailed studies depleting complement components reveal that, while disease is inhibited in the absence of a pathway, remyelination was also inhibited.

NK cells. The role of NK cells is controversial since depletion exacerbates EAE whereas in vitro NK cells damage oligodendrocytes and T cells. Their regulatory role and production of neuroprotective factors, e.g. brain-derived neuronal growth factor (BDNF), may explain the enhanced EAE when NK cells are depleted.

Mast cells generally aggravate EAE via BBB damage; however, EAE in mast cell-deficient (W(-sh)) mice is exacerbated (62) due to increased levels of proinflammatory cytokines, suggesting that mast cells are protective. In contrast, EAE in mast cell-deficient SJL mice is reduced and the animals develop relapsing disease (63).

T cells are present in the CNS of mice with EAE and have been reported to damage oligodendrocytes in vitro. Mice depleted of T cells develop less severe EAE probably due to reduced levels of proinflammatory cytokines and diminished expression of chemokines. However, depletion of T cells in B10.PL mice immunised with MBP causes a mild relapsing disease course compared to monophasic acute EAE.

Adaptive immunity

EAE is considered a paradigm CD4+ T cell-mediated disease since myelin-reactive T cells transfer disease. This hypothesis was challenged by the finding that myelin-reactive antibodies induce demyelination while Th2 T cells or CD8+ T cells also transfer disease.

CD4+ T cells. Detailed study of pathogenic T cells revealed a subpopulation of pathogenic Th1 T cells that express CXCR3 and CCR5, and secrete INF-γ and TNFα. EAE is exacerbated in mice deficient for INF-γ, TNFα, IFN-γR, and CXCR3. Activation of pathogenic T cells relies on IL-12 since blocking IL-12 inhibits EAE and IL-12 p35-deficient mice developed augmented EAE, while conversely mice lacking p40 are resistant. The p40 subunit is shared with IL-23 and IL-23-deficient mice are also resistant to EAE since IL-23 is necessary for maintenance of Th17 cells critical for EAE (64). In EAE proinflammatory cytokines associated with Th17 T cells correlate with damage in the CNS. Intriguingly, IL-9 is implicated in mediating pathogenic Th17-cell differentiation, since IL-9-deficient mice are resistant to EAE via inhibition of IL-17 (65).

CD8+ T cells. MHC class I is expressed in the CNS, including electrically silenced neurons, providing ideal targets for CD8+ T cells. CD8+ T cells are adjacent to transected neurites and neurons (66), while axonal damage is reduced in MHC class I-deficient mice. Once activated, CD8+ T cells express perforin, granzyme B, and Fas-L, all known to incite tissue damage. EAE is less severe in CD8+ T cell-deficient DBA/1 mice and CD8+ T cells transfer EAE, in which signs of ataxia and spasticity were observed (67). Also, humanised mice expressing MHC class I HLA-A*0301 and human CD8+ TCR-recognising PLP[45–53] develop low frequency of spontaneous disease. As well as pathogenic CD8+ T cells, it is thought their major effect in EAE is regulatory.

Regulatory T cells. Originally termed T suppressor cells, regulatory T cells (Tregs) are comprised of natural Tregs (nTreg), i.e. CD4+ CD25+ cells, or cells that can be induced to become Tregs, such as Th3, Tr1, CD8+ Treg, and NKT cells. While Tregs enter the CNS and proliferate, the balance of Tregs and T effector cells in the periphery regulates the chronicity, relapses, and remissions in EAE. Tregs are thought to exert their effect via cell-cell contact and production of inhibitory cytokines. In addition, modulation of co-stimulatory molecules via CTLA-4 and LFA-1 (CD11a) is demonstrated by studies in mice lacking LFA-1. These mice develop exacerbated EAE, due to decreased FoxP3+ Tregs and increased T effector cells (68). The decrease in Tregs was due to a defect in generation of nTregs in the thymus.

B cells and antibodies. Evidence for a role for humoral immunity in EAE comes from B cell depletion studies and transfer of pathogenic CNS-specific antibodies. B cell-deficient mice and depletion of B cells in EAE reveals that B cells play a role in activating the immune response via antigen presentation as well as secreting anti-inflammatory cytokines such as IL-10. B cells act by enhancing proliferation of MOG-specific T cells since depletion of B cells reduces T cell activation and production of IFN-γ and IL-17. The controversial role of B cells in EAE can be explained by their response to peptides or protein.

B cell-deficient C57BL/6 mice immunised with recombinant MOG do not develop EAE, while they are susceptible to MOG$^{35-55}$-induced EAE, probably because disease is dependent on antibodies to tertiary structures on MOG protein (69). However, mice deficient in the receptor for B cell activating factor (BAFF), critical for B cell survival, developed increased severity of EAE induced with MOG$^{35-55}$. Therapeutic strategies targeting B cells include the use of rituximab (anti-human CD20), which inhibits the development of clinical EAE in mice expressing human CD20, as it inhibits relapsing MS. That antibodies to MOG are important in disease is shown by adoptively transferring serum from animals immunised with recombinant MOG, or using pathogenic MOG monoclonal antibodies in mice (50). Antibodies to MOG are also crucial for EAE in marmosets as shown in tolerance studies. Here animals were protected against acute disease, but after administering MOG protein the animals developed a lethal demyelinating disorder associated with high levels of autoantibodies to MOG (70).

As well as pathogenic antibodies to myelin, antibodies to neuronal antigens isolated from MS patients are also pathogenic and exacerbate rat EAE due to increased axonal damage (57, 58).

Mutant and transgenic mouse models

Myelin mutant and transgenic mice have greatly aided our understanding of EAE. The effector mechanisms driving inflammation and demyelination, as well as remyelination and repair, can be dissected in myelin-deficient mice (Table 3.7), animals expressing T cell receptors to myelin proteins or human MHC molecules. In addition, mice over-expressing or lacking immune-related genes have helped uncover the role of cytokines and chemokines, B cells, and antibodies in EAE.

Myelin-deficient transgenic mice. EAE in MOG-deficient mice, or following immunisation with MOG-deficient myelin is significantly reduced thus stressing a key role of autoimmunity to MOG in EAE (14). In contrast, OMpg-deficient mice develop severe EAE. Yet another mouse, deficient in the myelin-associated protein, alpha B-crystallin, develops more severe EAE and enhanced oligodendrocyte apoptosis (71) indicating that this heat-shock protein may elicit a protective response.

Table 3.7 Animal mutants affecting CNS myelin

Name	Mutation	Clinical and pathological features
Shiverer mouse	Duplication and inversion of the gene encoding MBP	Shivering gait, early death, hypomyelination
Rumpshaker mouse	Mutation of PlP1 gene, misfolded PLP/DM20	Increased oligodendrocyte apoptosis
Quaking mouse	Reduction in QKI-5–7 in oligodendrocytes	Dysmyelination of CNS
Jimpy mouse	Point mutation in PLP gene	Severe CNS myelin deficiency and damage and oligodendrocyte apoptosis
Taiep rat	Defect in microtubule system and transport of myelin component	Tremor, ataxia, immobility episodes, epilepsy, and paralysis
Shaking dog	Decreased PLP gene expression, reduced PLP, MBP, CNPases, no effect on PNS	Tremor, seizures, and persistent neurological deficits, defects in oligodendrocytes development
OMgp null mice	Absence of gene for OMgp	Hypomyelination, severe EAE, slower nerve conduction velocity
MOG null mouse	Absence of gene for MOG	No phenotype but reduced severity of EAE

Transgenic models of autoimmunity. Spontaneous EAE is observed in mice generated to express T cell receptors (TCR) to MBP^{ac1-9}, PLP$^{139-151}$ or MOG$^{35-55}$, or humanised mice expressing TCRs for MBP$^{84-102}$ and HLA-DR2a (72), MOG and HLA-DR15, or MBP$^{111-129}$ HLA-DR4. The incidence of spontaneous EAE varies in the different transgenic mice; however, this variability depends also on the animal housing and husbandry. These findings point to a key role for infectious environments in activating pre-existing autoreactive T cells.

While EAE can be induced in B cell-deficient (μMT$-/-$) mice following immunisation with MBP or MOG peptides, recombinant MOG protein fails to induce disease (69). B cell-deficient mice do not recover from EAE due to a lack of IL-10, indicating that B cells fulfil a regulatory role in limiting disease. Transgenic mice expressing MOG$^{35-55}$ TCR (2D2 mice) crossed with mice expressing the MOG-specific immunoglobulin heavy chain (IgH^{MOG}) develop spontaneous EAE (73).

Chemokines and cytokines. In EAE chemokines and cytokines, crucial for cell recruitment and driving the autoimmune responses, have been dissected in transgenic mice. The impact of over-expression in the CNS on EAE is given in Table 3.8.

Over-expression of IFN-γ, IL-12, IL-6, IL-3, and TNFα in neurons, astrocytes, or oligodendrocytes enhances EAE. In the case of TNFα this depends on the expression of the receptor. These studies also reveal that cytokines and chemokines may be protective when expressed in the CNS, as shown with IL-12 p40 expression by astrocytes. Regarding chemokines and receptors, only transgenic mice expressing CCL21 or CXCL1 in oligodendrocytes developed neurological disease, albeit without demyelination, indicating that induction of chronic demyelinating EAE disease is multifactorial.

Table 3.8 Impact of over-expression of chemokines and cytokines in the CNS on EAE

Molecule	Promoter	Phenotype	Impact in EAE
TNFα	MBP	No phenotype	Augmented
TGF-β	GFAP	Motor disease	Augmented
IL-6	GFAP (cerebellum)		Severe ataxia yet no spinal cord damage
IL-12 p35/p40	GFAP	Ataxia, inflammation, T and NK cells, neurodegeneration	Enhanced
p40	GFAP	No phenotype	Reduced
CCL2	MBP	Increased recruitment of macrophages in the CNS. No clinical disease	Reduced

Table 3.9. Mice deficient for chemokines and cytokines: impact on EAE

Molecule	Impact on EAE
TNFα	Resistant to EAE due to ineffective priming of innate immune response
IFN-γ	Increased susceptibility to EAE
IL-1	IL-1α/β null mice develop reduced EAE and IFN-γ and IL-17-, IL-1α- or IL-1β-deficient mice develop EAE
IL-4	Severe EAE
IL-5	Deficient mice are susceptible. IL-5 thought to play a role in progression
IL-6	EAE resistant. Reduced T cell proliferation and endothelial activation
IL-10	Severe EAE associated with higher levels of Th1 cytokines. T cells adoptive transfer very severe EAE
IL-12	p35-deficient mice susceptible, p40-deficient mice are resistant
IL-17	Deletion of act1, required for IL-17 signaling, in astrocytes reduces EAE.
IL-23	p19 mice resistant to active EAE
GMF	Delayed and reduced severity
CXCL10	Lower threshold for disease induction
CCL2	Resistant to active EAE. T cells show decreased antigen-induced proliferation

The impact of cytokines and chemokines on EAE is better observed using deficient mice (Table 3.9) that, in general, support studies using blocking antibodies. However, deficiency may inhibit immune responses thus preventing the impact of manipulation on established disease. For this reason, conditional knock-out mice may provide more relevant information. In both examples, the activity or impact of the cytokine, and chemokines, on EAE depends on its location, the presence of the receptor, or ligand, as well as the model.

Guidelines for using, reporting, and reviewing EAE studies

EAE has greatly contributed to drug development in MS; however, therapies effective in EAE have not always translated to the clinic. The therapies that are in use in MS are glatiramer acetate, mitoxantrone, Tysabri, and Gilenya, and are described in detail in Chapter 7. The disparity between therapies that work in EAE and MS is in part due to the biology of animals and humans, but also to the quality and reporting of EAE studies that lack evidence of adoption of indicators of quality (74, 75, 76). Therefore, the ARRIVE (Animals in Research: Reporting In Vivo Experiments) guidelines were established to assist reporting of animal studies (74). To specifically address EAE studies, Vesterinen and colleagues (76) reviewed 1117 publications on EAE therapies concluding that few studies report measures of quality. Thus to improve conclusions drawn from EAE studies, and better translation to MS, a checklist incorporating the ARRIVE guidelines, principles of the 3Rs (Reduction, Refinement, and Replacement), and elements uncovered by Vesterinen's study (76) should be used (Table 3.10). These guidelines are currently under consideration by journals to also aid the review of EAE manuscripts. Several points in the checklist are self-explanatory and we only address those we consider crucial for EAE studies.

Materials and methods

Immunisation. Reproduction of studies relies on manuscripts providing sufficient information. While CFA is key for EAE induction few studies provide information on type and dose of mycobacterium, or the details of the antigen, for example the purity or chemical groups used to block functional groups.

Ethics. Within the EU, animals in research are protected by Directive 2010/63/EU, together with national and/or local legislations. EAE is a severe/substantial procedure, and where ethical review processes are not in place, it is crucial to adhere to the 3Rs principles. Studies should be refined, e.g. reducing the number of days animals are in the study once statistical analyses demonstrate an effect.

Monitoring. To limit bias, blinding should be used to avoid over-estimation of efficacy of treatments (76), e.g. coding the drug. The animal species and strain and the correct genetic nomenclature (http://www.informatics.jax.org/mgihome/nomen/) should be used. The term murine, meaning rat or mouse, should not be used. For drug studies animals should be randomised, e.g. equally distributing male and female animals.

Statistics. A power analysis is required before the start of the study to ensure sufficient numbers of animals in a group. Importantly, clinical EAE is non-linear (77) and non-parametric statistical analysis must be used. Thus, a Wilcoxon–Mann–Whitney U test and Kaplan–Meier test should be used and, when more than two groups are included, the Kruskal–Wallis test should be applied (77).

Pathology. As discussed, the pathology of EAE in rodents is primarily in the spinal cord. Brain lesions do not typically reflect clinical data in rodents and should not be used to assess or support differences in clinical disease between groups. While demyelination is a hallmark of MS, it is often presumed that primary demyelination occurs in EAE also. It is thus advised to perform double immunohistochemistry for neurofilament and myelin to establish whether areas of myelin loss are associated with or independent from axonal loss (78).

Table 3.10 Guidelines for reporting EAE studies

Item		Recommendation
Title	1	Accurate and concise description of study.
Abstract	2	Research objectives, animal species and strain, key methods, findings, and conclusions.
Introduction		
Background	3	a. With relevant references explain motivation and context of study. b. Experimental approach and rationale. c. Details of model and how this addresses objectives, and relevance to MS.
Hypothesis	4	Specific hypothesis and objectives.
Methods		
Ethical statement	5	a. Ethical review permissions, licences, guidelines for care and use of animals. b. Justify use of animals.
Study design	6	a. For each experiment give number of experimental and control groups. b. Discuss steps taken to randomise groups and assessment, i.e. blinding. c. Give experimental unit (e.g. single animal, group, or cage). For complex studies provide a timeline diagram.
Procedures	7	For each experiment and group, provide details of procedures. a. Dose, site, and route of drug administration, anaesthesia, surgical procedure, euthanasia. b. Details of specialist equipment and supplier. c. When, where, why.
Animals	8	a. Species, strain, sex, age, and weight ranges. b. Source, international nomenclature, genetic modification, genotype, health/immune status. c. For transgenic mice, give background of wild-type mice to alleviate breeding differences.
Housing and husbandry	9	a. Facility, e.g. SPF, cage or housing, bedding material, number of cage companions. b. Breeding programme, light/dark cycle, temperature, chow, access to food and water, environmental enrichment. c. Welfare-related assessments.
Sample size	10	a. Number of animals in each study and experimental group. b. Explain the number of animals, i.e. power analysis. c. Give number of replicates of each experiment.
Group allocation	11	a. Give full details of randomisation and matching. b. Describe order in which animals in experimental groups were treated and assessed.
Outcomes	12	Define outcomes, e.g. clinical, pathology, immunology, behavioural changes.

Table 3.10 (cont.)

Item		Recommendation
Statistics	13	a. Statistics – check that the test is appropriate. Clinical EAE scores are non-linear and require non-parametric analysis. b. Specify the unit of analysis for each dataset (e.g. single animal, single neuron). c. Describe methods used to assess whether data met assumptions of statistics.
Results		
Baseline data	14	Give health status of animals, e.g. weight, microbiological status, prior to treatment.
Numbers	15	a. Report absolute number of animals, e.g. 10/20, not 50%. b. Explain if data were not included. c. Explain if animals are kept in the study for longer than required.
Outcomes and estimation	16	a. Report measure of precision (e.g. standard error). b. Use statistics as in 13. Do not use area under the curve to compare groups.
Adverse events	17	a. Give details of important adverse events. b. Describe modifications of experimental protocols made to reduce adverse events.
Discussion		
Interpretation	18	a. Interpret results, referring to hypothesis, objectives, and published studies. b. Study limitations: potential bias, limitations of EAE, imprecision of results. c. Describe implications for the 3Rs.
Translation	19	Comment on relevance to MS, other diseases, human biology.
Funding	20	List funding sources including grant numbers.
Conflict of Interest (COI)	21	Disclose COI.

Results

Baseline data is recommended when out-bred animals are used since EAE may be influenced by infectious agents. The number of animals used should be reported in both the text and the figure legends to determine whether sufficient numbers have been used. For reproducibility the measure of deviation is essential. It is advised not to use 'area under the curve' to assess difference in EAE as the data may be misinterpreted. While seldom reported in EAE studies, adverse effects of therapies should also be noted as they could be very relevant as indicators of safety.

Regarding the discussions, funding, and conflicts of interests these are self-explanatory.

This guide should be used for executing and reporting EAE studies, or for reviewers of EAE manuscripts and grant applications.

Conclusions

EAE is an excellent model to examine inflammation in the CNS. Although not perfect, the models reflect many neurological and pathological characteristics of MS, yet still need refinement. The difference between EAE models and MS indicates that MS is not a straight-forward autoimmune disease targeting myelin, and thus the paradigm of aggressive CD4+ Th1 or Th17 cell responses to myelin antigens has undergone re-examination. The role of B cells and Tregs as well as the pathways leading to neurodegeneration have led to a paradigm shift in the thinking of MS. More appropriate models that reflect these features are still required. EAE and MS researchers are encouraged to be more critical of the existing EAE models and to become familiar with MS pathology and clinical disease to be fully aware of the disease they try to model. A critical approach to analysing and reporting EAE studies is crucial to allow effective translation to the clinic. When these points are considered there is a greater chance that EAE will help in uncovering the cause of MS and find an effective therapy.

Conflict of interest

The authors declare no conflict of interests.

Acknowledgements

Several of our studies on the topic have been financially supported by the Netherlands Foundation for MS Research and the Multiple Sclerosis Society of Great Britain and Northern Ireland.

References

1. Stuart, G. and Krikorian, K.S. (1930). A fatal neuro-paralytic accident of antirabies treatment. *Lancet* **1**, 1123–1125.

2. Rivers, T.M., Sprunt, D.H., and Berry, G.P. (1933). Observations on attempts to produce acute disseminated encephalomyelitis in monkeys. *J. Exp. Med.* **58**, 39–53.

3. Freund, J. and McDermott, K. (1942). Sensitisation to horse serum by means of adjuvants. *Proc. Soc. Exp. Biol.* **49**, 548–553.

4. Kabat, E.A., Wolf, A., and Bezer, A.E. (1947). The rapid production of acute disseminated encephalomyelitis in rhesus monkeys by injection of heterologous and homologous brain tissue with adjuvants. *J. Exp. Med.* **85**, 117–130

5. Libbey, J.E. and Fujinami, R.S. (2011). Experimental autoimmune encephalomyelitis as a testing paradigm for adjuvants and vaccines. *Vaccine* **29**, 3356–3362.

6. Smith, A.J., Liu, Y., Peng, H., *et al.* (2011). Comparison of a classical Th1 bacteria versus a Th17 bacteria as adjuvant in the induction of experimental autoimmune encephalomyelitis. *J. Neuroimmunol.* **237**, 33–38.

7. Andreasen, C., Powell, D.A., and Carbonetti, N.H. (2009). Pertussis toxin stimulates IL-17 production in response to *Bordetella pertussis* infection in mice. *PLoS ONE* **4**, e7079.

8. Richard, J.F., Roy, M., Audoy-Rémus, J., *et al.* (2011). Crawling phagocytes recruited in the brain vasculature after pertussis toxin exposure through IL6, ICAM1 and ITGαM. *Brain Pathol.* doi: 10.1111/j.1750-3639.2011.00490.x.

9. Tigno-Aranjuez, J.T., Jaini, R., Tuohy, V.K., Lehmann, P.V., and Tary-Lehmann, M. (2009). Encephalitogenicity of complete Freund's adjuvant relative to CpG is linked to induction of Th17 cells. *J. Immunol.* **183**, 5654–5661.

10. Staykova, M.A., Liñares, D., Fordham, S.A., Paridaen, J.T., and Willenborg, D.O.

(2008). The innate immune response to adjuvants dictates the adaptive immune response to autoantigens. *J. Neuropathol. Exp. Neurol.* **67**, 543–554.

11. Lorentzen J.C., Issazadeh S., Storch M., *et al.* (1995). Protracted, relapsing and demyelinating experimental autoimmune encephalomyelitis in DA rats immunized with syngeneic spinal cord and incomplete Freund's adjuvant. *J. Neuroimmunol.* **63**, 193–205.

12. Colover J. (1980). A new pattern of spinal-cord demyelination in guinea pigs with acute experimental allergic encephalomyelitis mimicking multiple sclerosis. *Br. J. Exp. Pathol.* **61**, 390–400.

13. Bielekova B., Goodwin B., Richert N., *et al.* (2000). Encephalitogenic potential of the myelin basic protein peptide (amino acids 83–99) in multiple sclerosis: results of a phase II clinical trial with an altered peptide ligand. *Nat. Med.* **6**, 1167–1175.

14. Smith, P.A., Heijmans, N., Ouwerling, B., *et al.* (2005). Native myelin oligodendrocyte glycoprotein promotes severe chronic neurological disease and demyelination in Biozzi ABH mice. *Eur. J. Immunol.* **35**, 1311–1319.

15. van Noort, J.M., van Sechel, A.C., Bajramovic, J.J., *et al.* (1995). The small heat-shock protein alpha B-crystallin as candidate autoantigen in multiple sclerosis. *Nature* **375**, 798–801.

16. van Noort, J.M., Bsibsi, M., Gerritsen, W.H., *et al.* (2010). AlphaB-crystallin is a target for adaptive immune responses and a trigger of innate responses in preactive multiple sclerosis lesions. *J. Neuropathol. Exp. Neurol.* **69**, 694–703.

17. Thoua, N, van Noort, J.M., Baker, D., *et al.* (2000). Encephalitogenic and immunological potential of the stress protein aB-crystallin (peptide 1–16) in Biozzi ABH (H-2Adq1) mice. *J. Neuroimmunol.* **104**, 47–57.

18. Huizinga, R., Heijmans, N., Schubert, P., *et al.* (2007). Immunization with neurofilament light protein induces spastic paresis and axonal degeneration in Biozzi ABH mice. *J. Neuropathol. Exp. Neurol.* **66**, 295–304.

19. Huizinga, R., Hintzen, R.Q., Assink, K., van Meurs, M., and Amor, S. (2009). T-cell responses to neurofilament light protein are part of a normal immune repertoire. *Int. Immunol.* **21**, 433–441.

20. Rosenmann, H., Grigoriadis, N., Karussis, D., *et al.* (2006). Tauopathy-like abnormalities and neurologic deficits in mice immunized with neuronal tau protein. *Arch. Neurol.* **63**, 1459–1467.

21. Al-Izki, S., Pryce, G., O'Neill, J.K., *et al.* (2011). Practical guide to the induction of relapsing progressive experimental autoimmune encephalomyelitis in the Biozzi ABH mouse. *Multiple Sclerosis and Related Disorders* **1**, 29–38.

22. Baker, D., O'Neill, J.K., Gschmeissner, S.E., *et al.* (1990). Induction of chronic relapsing experimental allergic encephalomyelitis in Biozzi mice. *J. Neuroimmunol.* **28**, 261–270.

23. Amor, S., Smith, P.A., Hart, B., and Baker, D. (2005). Biozzi mice: of mice and human neurological diseases. *J. Neuroimmunol.* **165**, 1–10.

24. Hampton, D.W., Anderson, J., Pryce, G., *et al.* (2008). An experimental model of secondary progressive multiple sclerosis that shows regional variation in gliosis, remyelination, axonal and neuronal loss. *J. Neuroimmunol.* **201**, 200–211

25. Amor S., O'Neill, J.K., Morris, M.M., *et al.* (1996). Encephalitogenic epitopes of myelin basic protein, proteolipid protein and myelin oligodendrocyte protein for EAE induction in Biozzi ABH (H-2Adq1) mice share an amino acid motif. *J. Immunol.* **156**, 3000–3008.

26. Morris-Downes, M.M., McCormack, K., Baker, D., *et al.* (2002). Encephalitogenic and immunogenic potential of myelin-associated glycoprotein (MAG), oligodendrocyte-specific glycoprotein (OSP) and 2',3'-cyclic nucleotide 3'-phosphodiesterase (CNPase) in ABH and SJL mice. *J. Neuroimmunol.* **122**, 20–33.

27. Huizinga, R., Gerritsen, W., Heijmans, N., and Amor, S. (2008). Axonal loss and gray

matter pathology as a direct result of autoimmunity to neurofilaments. *Neurobiol. Dis.* **32**, 461–470.

28. Amor, S., Baker, D., Groome, N., and Turk, J.L. (1993). Identification of a major encephalitogenic epitope of proteolipid protein (Residues 56–70) for the induction of experimental allergic encephalomyelitis in Biozzi AB/H mice. *J. Immunol.* **150**, 5666–5672.

29. Amor, S., Groome, N., Linington, C., *et al.* (1994). Identification of epitopes of myelin oligodendrocyte glycoprotein for the induction of experimental allergic encephalomyelitis in SJL and Biozzi AB/H mice. *J. Immunol.* **153**, 4349–4356.

30. Levine, S. and Sowinski, R. (1973). Hyperacute allergic encephalomyelitis: a localized form produced by passive transfer and pertussis vaccine. *Am. J. Pathol.* **73**, 247–260.

31. Swanborg, R.H. (2001). Experimental autoimmune encephalomyelitis in the rat: lessons in T-cell immunology and autoreactivity. *Immunol. Rev.* **184**, 129–135.

32. Raine, C.S., Traugott, U., and Stone, S.H. (1978). Chronic relapsing experimental allergic encephalomyelitis: CNS plaque development in unsuppressed and suppressed animals. *Acta Neuropathol.* **43**, 43–53.

33. Gambi, D., Di Cesare, N., Di Trapani, G., Macchi, G., and Sbriccoli, A. (1989). Experimental allergic encephalomyelitis in guinea pig: variability of response to intradermal emulsion injection. *Ital. J. Neurol. Sci.* **10**, 33–41.

34. Genain, C.P. and Hauser, S.L. (1996). Allergic encephalomyelitis in common marmosets: pathogenesis of a multiple sclerosis-like lesion. *Methods* **10**, 420–434.

35. Jagessar, S.A., Smith, P.A., Blezer, E., *et al.* (2008). Autoimmunity against myelin oligodendrocyte glycoprotein is dispensable for the initiation although essential for the progression of chronic encephalomyelitis in common marmosets. *J. Neuropathol. Exp. Neurol.* **67**, 326–340.

36. van Lambalgen, R. and Jonker, M. (1987). Experimental allergic encephalomyelitis in rhesus monkeys: I. Immunological parameters in EAE resistant and susceptible rhesus monkeys. *Clin. Exp. Immunol.* **68**, 100–107.

37. Shaw, C.M., Alvord, E.C. Jr., and Hruby, S. (1988). Chronic remitting-relapsing experimental allergic encephalomyelitis induced in monkeys with homologous myelin basic protein. *Ann. Neurol.* **24**, 738–748.

38. Bajramovic, J.J., Brok, H.P., Ouwerling, B., *et al.* (2008). Oligodendrocyte-specific protein is encephalitogenic in rhesus macaques and induces specific demyelination of the optic nerve. *Eur. J. Immunol.* **38**, 1452–1464.

39. Brown, A.M., and McFarlin, D.E. (1981). Relapsing experimental allergic encephalomyelitis in the SJL/J mouse. *Lab. Invest.* **45**, 278–284.

40. Zamvil, S., Nelson, P., Trotter, J., *et al.* (1985). T-cell clones specific for myelin basic protein induce chronic relapsing paralysis and demyelination. *Nature* **317**, 355–358.

41. Tuohy, V.K., Lu, Z., Sobel, R.A., Laursen, R.A., and Lees, M.B. (1989). Identification of an encephalitogenic determinant of myelin proteolipid protein for SJL mice. *J. Immunol.* **142**, 1523–1527.

42. Mendel, I., Kerlero de Rosbo, N., and Ben-Nun, A. (1995). A myelin oligodendrocyte glycoprotein peptide induces typical chronic experimental autoimmune encephalomyelitis in H-2b mice: fine specificity and T cell receptor V beta expression of encephalitogenic T cells. *Eur. J. Immunol.* **25**, 1951–1959.

43. Teuscher, C., Bunn, J.Y., Fillmore, P.D., *et al.* (2004). Gender, age, and season at immunization uniquely influence the genetic control of susceptibility to histopathological lesions and clinical signs of experimental allergic encephalomyelitis: implications for the genetics of multiple sclerosis. *Am. J. Pathol.* **165**, 1593–1602.

44. Ditamo, Y., Degano, A.L., Maccio, D.R., Pistoresi-Palencia, M.C., and Roth, G.A.

(2005). Age-related changes in the development of experimental autoimmune encephalomyelitis. *Immunol. Cell Biol.* **83**, 75–82.

45. Yoshimura, T., Kunishita, T., Sakai, K., *et al.* (1985). Chronic experimental allergic encephalomyelitis in guinea pigs induced by proteolipid protein. *J. Neurol. Sci.* **69**, 47–58.

46. Pomeroy, I.M., Jordan, E.K., Frank, J.A., Matthews, P.M., and Esiri, M.M. (2010). Focal and diffuse cortical degenerative changes in a marmoset model of multiple sclerosis. *Mult. Scler.* **16**, 537–548.

47. Kerlero de Rosbo, N., Brok, H.P., Bauer, J., *et al.* (2000). Rhesus monkeys are highly susceptible to experimental autoimmune encephalomyelitis induced by myelin oligodendrocyte glycoprotein: characterisation of immunodominant T- and B-cell epitopes. *J. Neuroimmunol.* **110**, 83–96.

48. Bartanusz, V., Jezova, D., Alajajian, B., and Digicaylioglu, M. (2011). The blood-spinal cord barrier: morphology and clinical implications. *Ann. Neurol.* **70**, 194–206.

49. Amor, S., Puentes, F., Baker, D., and van der Valk, P. (2010) Inflammation in neurodegenerative diseases. *Immunology* **129**, 154–169.

50. Morris-Downes, M.M., Smith, P.A., Rundle, J.L., *et al.* (2002). Pathological and regulatory effects of anti-myelin antibodies in experimental allergic encephalomyelitis in mice. *J. Neuroimmunol.* **125**, 114–124.

51. Girolamo, F., Ferrara, G., Strippoli, M., *et al.* (2011). Cerebral cortex demyelination and oligodendrocyte precursor response to experimental autoimmune encephalomyelitis. *Neurobiol. Dis.* **43**, 678–689.

52. Harris, R.A. and Amor, S. (2011). Sweet and sour – oxidative and carbonyl stress in neurological disorders. *CNS Neurol. Disord. Drug Targets* **10**, 82–107.

53. Parratt, J.D. and Prineas, J.W. (2010). Neuromyelitis optica: a demyelinating disease characterized by acute destruction and regeneration of perivascular astrocytes. *Mult. Scler.* **16**, 1156–1172.

54. Hövelmeyer, N., Hao, Z., Kranidioti, K., *et al.* (2005). Apoptosis of oligodendrocytes via Fas and TNF-R1 is a key event in the induction of experimental autoimmune encephalomyelitis. *J. Immunol.* **175**, 5875–5884.

55. Mi, S., Lee, X., Hu, Y., *et al.* (2011). Death receptor 6 negatively regulates oligodendrocyte survival, maturation and myelination. *Nat. Med.* **17**, 816–821.

56. Mangiardi, M., Crawford, D.K., Xia, X., *et al.* (2011). An animal model of cortical and callosal pathology in multiple sclerosis. *Brain Pathol.* **21**, 263–278.

57. Mathey, E.K., Derfuss, T., Storch, M.K., *et al.* (2007). Neurofascin as a novel target for autoantibody-mediated axonal injury. *J. Exp. Med.* **204**, 2363–2372.

58. Derfuss, T., Parikh, K., Velhin, S., *et al.* (2009). Contactin-2/TAG-1-directed autoimmunity is identified in multiple sclerosis patients and mediates gray matter pathology in animals. *Proc. Natl. Acad. Sci. U.S.A.* **106**, 8302–8307.

59. Toft-Hansen, H., Füchtbauer, L., and Owens, T. (2011). Inhibition of reactive astrocytosis in established experimental autoimmune encephalomyelitis favors infiltration by myeloid cells over T cells and enhances severity of disease. *Glia* **59**, 166–176.

60. Bajramovic, J.J. (2011). Regulation of innate immune responses in the central nervous system. *CNS Neurol. Disord. Drug Targets.* **10**, 4–24.

61. Hoarau, J.J., Krejbich-Trotot, P., Jaffar-Bandjee, M.C., *et al.* (2011). Activation and control of CNS innate immune responses in health and diseases: a balancing act finely tuned by neuroimmune regulators (NIReg). *CNS Neurol. Disord. Drug Targets.* **10**, 25–43.

62. Li, H., Nourbakhsh, B., Safavi, F., *et al.* (2011). Kit (W-sh) mice develop earlier and more severe experimental autoimmune encephalomyelitis due to absence of immune suppression. *J. Immunol.* **187**, 274 -282.

63. Sayed, B.A., Walker, M.E., and Brown, M.A. (2011). Cutting edge: mast cells

regulate disease severity in a relapsing-remitting model of multiple sclerosis. *J. Immunol.* **186**, 3294–3298.

64. Zepp, J., Wu, L., and Li, X. (2011). IL-17 receptor signaling and T helper 17-mediated autoimmune demyelinating disease. *Trends Immunol.* **32**, 232–239.

65. Batoulis, H., Addicks, K., and Kuerten, S. (2010). Emerging concepts in autoimmune encephalomyelitis beyond the CD4/T(H)1 paradigm. *Ann. Anat.* **92**, 179–193.

66. Vogt, J., Paul, F., Aktas, O., *et al.* (2009). Lower motor neuron loss in multiple sclerosis and experimental autoimmune encephalomyelitis. *Ann. Neurol.* **66**, 310–322.

67. Sun, D., Whitaker, J.N., Huang, Z., *et al.* (2001). Myelin antigen-specific CD8+ T cells are encephalitogenic and produce severe disease in C57BL/6 mice. *J. Immunol.* **166**, 7579–7587.

68. Gültner, S., Kuhlmann, T., Hesse, A., *et al.* (2010). Reduced Treg frequency in LFA-1-deficient mice allows enhanced T effector differentiation and pathology in EAE. *Eur. J. Immunol.* **40**, 3403–3412.

69. Lyons, J.A., San, M., Happ, M.P., Cross, A.H. (1999). B cells are critical to induction of experimental allergic encephalomyelitis by protein but not by a short encephalitogenic peptide. *Eur. J. Immunol.* **29**, 3432–3439.

70. Genain, C.P., Abel, K., Belmar, N., *et al.* (1996). Late complications of immune deviation therapy in a nonhuman primate. *Science* **274**, 2054–2057.

71. Ousman, S.S., Tomooka, B.H., van Noort, J.M., *et al.* (2007). Protective and therapeutic role for alphaB-crystallin in autoimmune demyelination. *Nature* **448**, 474–479.

72. Ellmerich, S., Takacs, K., Mycko, M., *et al.* (2004). Disease-related epitope spread in a humanized T cell receptor transgenic model of multiple sclerosis. *Eur. J. Immunol.* **34**, 1839–1848.

73. Krishnamoorthy, G., Lassmann, H., Wekerle, H., and Holz, A. (2006). Spontaneous opticospinal encephalomyelitis in a double-transgenic mouse model of autoimmune T cell/B cell cooperation. *J. Clin. Invest.* **116**, 2385–2392.

74. Kilkenny, C., Browne, W.J., Cuthill, I.C., Emerson, M., and Altman, D.G. (2010). Improving bioscience research reporting: the ARRIVE guidelines for reporting animal research. *PLoS Biol.* **8**, e1000412.

75. Baker, D. and Amor, S. (2010). Quality control of experimental autoimmune encephalomyelitis. *Mult. Scler.* **16**, 1025–1027

76. Vesterinen, H.M., Sena, E.S., Ffrench-Constant, C., *et al.* (2010). Improving the translational hit of experimental treatments in multiple sclerosis. *Mult. Scler.* **16**, 1044–1055.

77. Fleming, K.K., Bovaird, J.A., Moiser, M.C., *et al.* (2005). Statistical analysis of data from studies on experimental autoimmune encephalomyelitis. *J. Neuroimmunol.* **170**, 71–84.

78. Baker, D., Gerritsen, W., Rundle, J., and Amor, S. (2011). Critical appraisal of animal models of multiple sclerosis. *Mult. Scler.* **17**, 647–657.

Chapter 4

Immunology of MS

Jean M. Fletcher and Kingston H.G. Mills

Introduction

MS is an autoimmune disease of the central nervous system of unknown etiology and with no known cure. It is thought to be triggered in genetically susceptible individuals in response to environmental factors. There is strong evidence that the immune system plays a key role in the pathogenesis of MS. The strongest genetic association with MS is with MHC class II genes, the products of which present antigen to CD4+ T cells. Infiltrating immune cells are found in the CNS of patients with MS and immunosuppressive drugs that prevent lymphocyte migration or function are moderately effective therapies for relapsing–remitting MS (RRMS). However, despite many years of research, some of the key questions remain unanswered and a cure remains elusive. Nonetheless, there has recently been much progress in understanding the underlying immunological dysfunction and identifying novel therapeutic targets, with the result that a number of more specifically targeted therapies are now in pre-clinical development or are in clinical trials. In this chapter we will review the current knowledge on the role of the immune system in MS.

Tolerance and autoimmunity

The primary function of the immune system is to defend against infection by pathogens. This requires an ability to recognise pathogen antigens specifically, as well as effector mechanisms to eliminate the infectious agent. However, it is also important for the immune system not to over-respond to pathogens, which can lead to immunopathology, and to avoid reacting against self antigens (Figure 4.1). The prevention of immune responses to self antigens is maintained by both central and peripheral tolerance mechanisms. Central tolerance is controlled in the thymus and bone marrow, where high-affinity self-reactive T and B cells, respectively, are deleted. Self-reactive T and B cells with low or intermediate affinity escape this process and are controlled by peripheral tolerance, which is mediated by different mechanisms, including antigen segregation, anergy induction, and the suppressive effects of regulatory T cells. A failure in immunological tolerance can result in the development of autoimmune diseases in genetically susceptible individuals. A number of factors can contribute to the development of autoimmunity. These include molecular mimicry, which can occur in the context of infection or tumours, when there is cross-reactivity with a self antigen. Alternatively, infection injury or trauma can provide or

The Biology of Multiple Sclerosis, ed Gregory J. Atkins, Sandra Amor, Jean M. Fletcher and Kingston H.G. Mills. Published by Cambridge University Press. © Gregory J. Atkins, Sandra Amor, Jean M. Fletcher and Kingston H.G. Mills 2012.

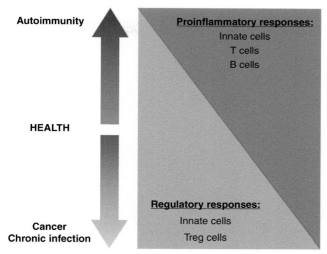

Autoimmunity

Proinflammatory responses:
Innate cells
T cells
B cells

HEALTH

Regulatory responses:
Innate cells
Treg cells

Cancer
Chronic infection

Figure 4.1. Dysregulation of immune responses in autoimmunity. In the healthy immune system, proinflammatory responses which are required to fight infection and prevent tumours are balanced by regulatory responses. Regulatory responses, including innate mechanisms and regulatory T cells, are required to prevent immunopathology and maintain tolerance to self antigens. In autoimmunity, the balance of the immune system is shifted in favour of inflammation. In contrast, during chronic infection and cancers, the immune system may be unable to mount an effective proinflammatory response in the face of an overly regulatory environment.

provoke the release of danger signals that promote innate immune responses that drive pathogenic autoantigen-specific T cells. In the case of MS the trigger is unknown, however infections have been implicated (discussed in more detail in Chapter 6).

Pathogenesis of MS

It is generally presumed that RRMS is triggered when autoreactive myelin-specific CD4 T cells are activated in the peripheral lymphoid organs by an unknown trigger (Figure 4.2). T cells specific for myelin antigens can be detected in healthy controls as well as in MS patients (1). Therefore, it is not the presence of these cells per se that causes MS, rather, it is thought that the self-reactive myelin-specific T cells are inappropriately activated or inadequately regulated in MS patients. Activated T cells express the appropriate array of molecules that allow them to leave the lymph node, enter the circulation, and home to the CNS where they pass through the blood–brain barrier in a two-step process. To enter the CNS parenchyma, T cells must first traverse the tight junctions between the endothelial cells lining the blood vessels into the perivascular space, and then cross the glia limitans, which is formed by a basement membrane and astrocyte end-feet. Secretion of matrix metalloproteinases (MMP) by migrating T cells permeabilises the basal lamina. After entering the CNS and encountering their cognate myelin antigen, presented by either CNS-resident or infiltrating APC, autoreactive myelin-specific T cells undergo clonal expansion and secrete cytokines. The release of cytokines by re-activated T cells activates resident micoglia, further permeabilises the blood–brain barrier, and recruits other inflammatory leucocytes via chemotaxis. Infiltrating monocytes, NK cells, and activated T and B cells all contribute to the inflammatory cascade via cytotoxicity, production of cytokines, antibody, proteases, and toxic mediators,

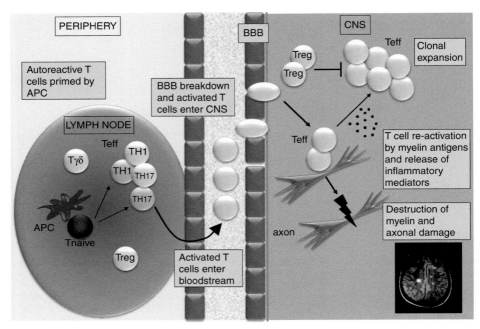

Figure 4.2. Steps involved in the development of RRMS. It is thought RRMS is triggered in susceptible individuals when autoreactive T cells specific for myelin antigens are activated in the peripheral lymphoid organs, possibly in the context of infection. The activated myelin-specific T cells enter the bloodstream and traffic to and enter the CNS. Breakdown of the BBB occurs, allowing recruitment of other inflammatory cells into the CNS. T cells entering the CNS encounter their cognate myelin antigens and become re-activated by local APC. T cells expand and release inflammatory mediators which help to recruit other immune cells to the site of inflammation. Activation of local microglial cells and infiltrating cells results in production of proteases, glutamate, reactive oxygen species, and other cytotoxic agents which promote myelin breakdown. Damage to the myelin sheath surrounding axons is followed by axonal damage and neurological impairment.

such as ROS and glutamate. The resulting destruction of the myelin sheath surrounding axons is one of the key pathological features of MS. The myelin sheath insulates axons and provides quicker nerve conduction, thus demyelination leads to slowing or even complete blockage of nerve conduction and demyelinated axons are left susceptible to damage by inflammatory mediators and cytotoxic cells. The acute inflammatory lesions that occur during RRMS are characterised by breakdown of the blood–brain barrier, infiltration of CD4 and CD8 αβ T cells, γδ T cells, B cells, NK cells, and macrophages. CD4 T cells are not a major component of inflammatory lesions and are outnumbered by CD8 T cells, suggesting that although they are important in initiating autoimmune inflammation in MS, they make less of a contribution to demyelination and axonal damage. Axonal loss begins in active lesions during early RRMS and there is gradual accrual of axonal loss and disability with time. However, progressive neurodegeneration continues during SPMS, where there is generally an absence of active new lesions. In contrast to the active focal lesions that occur mainly in the white matter during RRMS, progressive forms of MS are characterised by widespread demyelination in the cortex as well as diffuse degenerative changes throughout the entire white and grey matter and brain atrophy (2). Chronic microglial activation and release of toxic mediators, mitochondrial dysfunction, and disturbances in sodium channels are all thought to play a role in the progression of MS (3).

Myelin antigens

Much of the early research on the immunology of MS focused on the specificity of pathogenic CD4 T cells. These are generally thought to be specific for myelin antigens, since demyelination is the hallmark of MS pathogenesis, and EAE is induced by immunisation with myelin peptides; however, this may be an oversimplification. A number of immunodominant epitopes from myelin basic protein (MBP), myelin oligodendrocyte protein (MOG), and phospholipid protein (PLP) were identified early on (1, 4, 5). These peripheral autoreactive myelin-specific T cells are thought to be low avidity cells that escaped deletion in the thymus. Although myelin-specific CD4 T cells could also be detected in healthy controls, many studies showed increased or altered T cell responses to particular myelin epitopes in MS patients (4, 6–11). The specificity of the oligoclonal antibodies that are often found in the CSF of patients with RRMS has been difficult to identify, although MOG-specific antibodies have been reported in paediatric MS (12). In the EAE model immunisation with a MOG peptide results in the generation of MOG-specific T cell responses. However, as myelin is damaged, it is thought that the exposure of alternative myelin epitopes results in 'epitope spreading' where there is a gradual broadening of the repertoire of encephalitogenic T cells (13, 14). A similar process may occur in MS (15), and it has been suggested that this might account for the pattern of relapse and remission, where responses against new epitopes could trigger a relapse.

Progression of MS

Over 80% of MS patients present with the RR form of the disease, and after a variable length of time the majority progress to a secondary progressive (SP) course. RRMS is characterised by intermittent acute episodes or relapses during which patients experience symptoms that resolve completely or partially within a few days. Relapses are accompanied by an influx of inflammatory cells into the CNS and breakdown of the blood–brain barrier. There is a gradual accrual of baseline disability over time in RRMS, as full function is not always regained after relapses. The SP form of the disease usually follows on from RRMS after a variable number of years and is characterised by a steady decline in neurological function in the relative absence of relapses (Figure 4.3). Approximately 10% of MS patients exhibit a primary progressive (PP) course, where there is a steady decline in function from the start, in the absence of relapses.

Much of the research on the immunology of MS has focused on the role of the adaptive immune system, particularly CD4 T cells, since autoreactive myelin-specific CD4 T cells are thought to be responsible for initiating disease. Indeed, the currently licensed first-line treatments for MS have been shown to have anti-inflammatory effects on T cells. However, while these therapies have efficacy against RRMS, they are ineffective in treating the progressive forms of the disease, and this represents one of the biggest challenges in MS. Furthermore, there is no clear evidence that current treatments for RRMS will prevent or even slow down the transition to SPMS. Thus, clearly different disease processes are involved in mediating SPMS versus RRMS. While RRMS is characterised by active inflammatory plaques in the CNS, the progressive phase of MS is characterised by neurodegenerative processes

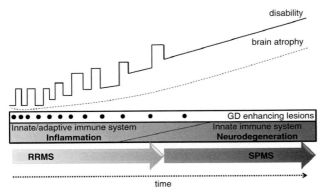

Figure 4.3. The disease course in MS. RRMS is characterised by active gadolinium enhancing lesions and relapses. RRMS is driven by T cells and other components of the adaptive and innate immune systems, and is responsive to anti-inflammatory therapy. After a variable number of years the majority of patients with RRMS progress to SPMS, which is characterised by a relative absence of new lesions but accumulating disability. SPMS does not respond to anti-inflammatory therapy, and it is thought that the innate immune system contributes to the ongoing neurodegeneration. The progression of MS is also associated with brain atrophy.

involving chronic activation of innate immune cells in the CNS. The contribution of the innate and adaptive arms of the immune system to MS will be discussed below.

Role of the innate immune system

The innate immune system represents a crucial first line of defence against infection, but also directs the induction of the adaptive immune response. Innate cells recognise pathogen-derived antigens via a system of invariant receptors, called pathogen recognition receptors (PRRs), which unlike those of the adaptive immune system do not undergo gene rearrangement and have no immunological memory. PRRs include toll-like receptors (TLRs), Nod-like receptors (NLRs), and RIG-I-like receptors (RLRs), which respond to pathogen-associated molecular patterns (PAMPs) as well as endogenous stress signals (damage-associated molecular patterns (DAMPs)).

Although MS has been thought of as a primarily T cell-mediated autoimmune disease, cells of the innate immune system play an important role in disease, by acting as APC for T cells, providing a source of cytokines that shape adaptive immune responses and contribute to inflammatory pathology during RRMS. Furthermore it is now thought that chronic activation of innate cells in the CNS contributes to the progressive disability that occurs during SPMS (16, 17; Figure 4.3).

Dendritic cells

Dendritic cells (DCs) are considered to be the professional APC of the immune system, due to their specialist ability to prime naïve T cells and orchestrate the differentiation of naïve T cells. DCs can be broadly divided into myeloid DCs (mDCs), which are thought to have a pathogenic role, and plasmacytoid (pDCs), which may play a more regulatory role in EAE and MS (18). In the EAE model, disease can be adoptively transferred by mDCs primed with myelin antigens. Aside from their important role in T cell priming in the periphery, peripheral mDCs also accumulate and present antigens to pathogenic T cells within the CNS (19). The phenotype and function of mDCs is altered in MS. Monocyte-derived DCs from RRMS patients secreted higher levels of IL-23 (20), and circulating DCs with an activated phenotype and higher expression of IL-12 were observed in patients with SPMS compared with those with RRMS or controls (21). In contrast pDCs from MS patients were reported to have an immature regulatory phenotype (22). These studies suggest that mDCs and pDCs play a role in regulating immune responses during both RR and SPMS.

Microglial cells and macrophages

Resident microglial cells are the most common immune cells in the CNS. During MS and EAE monocytes infiltrate the CNS and differentiate into macrophages, which are indistinguishable from the resident microglial cells. A recent study showed that although infiltrating monocytes were essential for the pathogenesis of EAE, they disappeared upon remission and therefore do not contribute to the resident microglial pool (23). Microglial cells express TLR, MHC class II, and co-stimulatory molecules and are capable of multiple immune functions, such as phagocytosis, cytokine secretion, and antigen presentation (24). Microglial cells are considered to be the resident APC of the CNS, where they present antigens to autoreactive T cells. This is important in initiating and maintaining autoimmune responses in the CNS (24). Furthermore microglial activation in EAE contributes directly to CNS damage through several mechanisms, including the production of proinflammatory cytokines, matrix metalloproteinases, and free radicals (24). Chronic microglial activation is a feature of progressive MS, and is thought to contribute to neurodegeneration (16).

Natural killer cells and natural killer T cells

NK cells form an important part of the early antiviral response and anti-tumour responses, by secreting antiviral cytokines, activating DCs and cytotoxicity. NK cells are present in MS lesions (25), and both pathogenic and protective functions have been ascribed to different populations of NK cells during MS. CD56^{bright} NK cells secrete a range of regulatory cytokines, while CD56^{dim} NK cells are more cytotoxic (26). NK cells can potentially contribute to CNS damage via cytotoxicity towards microglial cells, astrocytes, and oligodendrocytes. Furthermore, proinflammatory NK cells secreting IL-17 and IFN-γ were recently found to be enriched in the CSF from MS patients (27). However, a number of studies have also suggested a more protective role for NK cells during MS and EAE (28). Decreased frequencies of NK cells have been associated with MS and clinically isolated syndrome (CIS) (29). Furthermore, the frequency of CD56^{bright} NK cells was increased after therapy with daclizumab and IFN-β (30, 31), and correlated with response to IFN-β (31). These regulatory effects of CD56^{bright} NK cells may be mediated via the secretion of anti-inflammatory cytokines or via cytotoxicity of autoreactive T cells.

Natural killer T (NKT) cells are a small population of thymus-derived T cells that are restricted by the non-classical MHC class I molecule CD1d. NKT cells are thought to have a protective role in MS; NKT cells are found at a lower frequency with defective cytokine production in MS patients (reviewed in (32)). Furthermore, like NK cells, there is an increase in frequency and function of NKT cells after immunomodulatory therapy (33).

$\gamma\delta$ T cells

T cells recognise non-MHC restricted antigens via their invariant $\gamma\delta$ T cell receptors, and are thought to provide a first line of defence against infection, especially at mucosal sites, through the production of IFN-$\gamma\delta$. T cells directly recognise ligands induced by stress, inflammation or infection, including non-classical MHC class I molecules, such as MIC A and MIC B, non-peptide antigens, alkylamines, phosphoantigens, and heat-shock proteins. T cells can act as a source of innate cytokine and thus have the potential to influence adaptive immune responses.

For the last 10–15 years T cells have been thought to play a role in both MS and EAE. Clonally expanded γδ T cells are present in acute MS brain lesions (34) and in the CSF of recent onset MS patients (35), suggesting that γδ T cells contribute to CNS inflammation. However, in the EAE model, both pathogenic (36–40) and protective (41–43) roles have been attributed to γδ T cells. It has recently been shown that IL-17 can be produced by γδ T cells (44, 45), and recent data from our laboratory has shown that IL-17-producing γδ T cells are present at high frequency in the CNS of mice with EAE (46). Furthermore, disease was less severe in $Tcrd^{-/-}$ mice, supporting a pathogenic role for γδ T cells. MOG-specific IL-17 production by conventional γδ T cells was reduced in $Tcrd^{-/-}$ mice and this was consistent with the demonstration that γδ T cell-derived IL-17 and IL-21 promoted further IL-17 production by CD4+ T cells (46). γδ T cells were shown to produce IL-17 in response to IL-1 and IL-23 in the absence of TCR engagement, and these cells increased susceptibility to EAE. Thus in addition to being an important source of IL-17 early in the EAE disease course, γδ T cells also served to amplify IL-17 production by CD4+ γδ T cells (46). Overall, the consensus from the various studies suggests a pathogenic role for γδ T cells in EAE, particularly early in the disease course, although they may also have a regulatory role during disease resolution in some models (42, 43, 46). IL-17-producing γδ cells have not yet been demonstrated in MS. Heat-shock proteins have been implicated as the target of autoreactive γδ T cells in MS, since heat-shock proteins are expressed in the CNS (34) and γδ T cells specific for heat-shock proteins have been isolated from MS patients (47). Furthermore, γδ T cells expressing CD16 were found to be elevated during progressive MS (48) and capable of lysing oligodendrocytes (49).

The contribution of innate immunity during different stages of MS and EAE

In the EAE model, mice are immunised with a myelin peptide together with complete Freund's adjuvant, containing killed *Mycobacterium tuberculosis* (Mtb). The Mtb component provides innate signals which are essential to break down tolerance to the myelin self antigen, and disease is not induced in the absence of Mtb. Mtb contains various TLRs and TLR ligands, which innate signaling pathways have shown to be essential for induction of autoimmune inflammation. $Myd88^{-/-}$ (a signaling molecule downstream from TLRs and IL-1) mice are resistant to EAE induction (50). A recent study also indicates a novel role for commensal gut flora, which, in the absence of pathogenic agents, were essential in triggering RR EAE (51). In MS, it has long been suspected that infection, together with other environmental factors, is responsible for triggering disease. Infection has the potential to break tolerance and trigger autoimmunity by molecular mimicry, bystander activation, or triggering of PRR on innate cells to provide the appropriate cytokine milieu for the generation of pathogenic T cells. However, the precise mechanism through which infections (discussed in Chapter 6) might trigger MS is still unknown, but it is likely that the innate immune system is involved. It is also possible that trauma, cell death, or cell stress could trigger autoimmunity via the release of DAMPs and the development of sterile inflammation.

TLR signaling appears to be necessary for the effector phase as well as induction of EAE. Various TLRs are expressed in the CNS during MS (52) and EAE, but TLR7 and TLR9 in particular are highly expressed during the peak of disease in the EAE model (50). Furthermore, TLR9 signaling in the CNS was shown to be required for the effector phase of disease. Since the CNS is normally a sterile environment, this may suggest the involvement of endogenous TLR9 ligands in promoting CNS inflammation (50). Infections have been implicated in triggering relapses during RRMS, possibly as a result of bystander activation (53). Activation of innate cells by DAMPs in response to cellular stress or death could potentially also precipitate relapse and contribute to disease progression in MS (54). On the other hand, innate immune signaling can also have a protective effect, since TLR3 stimulation ameliorated EAE via the induction of endogenous IFN-β (55).

During progressive MS, the occurrence of relapses and new lesions subsides. However disability continues to accumulate due to ongoing neurodegeneration. PP and SP MS are refractory to the anti-inflammatory therapeutic strategies that are effective in RRMS, indicating important differences in the pathological processes involved in the different forms of MS. In contrast to the active focal lesions that occur mainly in the white matter during RRMS, progressive forms of MS are characterised by widespread demyelination in the cortex as well as diffuse degenerative changes throughout the entire white and grey matter and brain atrophy (2). The neurodegenerative processes underlying SPMS are not yet well understood, but are likely to be mediated or supported by innate immune cells within the CNS (17, 56). CNS-resident innate cells, such as microglia and macrophages, are chronically activated during progressive MS, and produce toxic intermediates, such as glutamate, ROS, and NO (57). Once axons are demyelinated, they are more susceptible to damage by such soluble factors. Chronic activation of innate cells by endogenous DAMPs could perpetuate neurodegeneration during progressive MS. Consistent with this idea, serum concentrations of oxidised derivatives of cholesterol (15-HC), a breakdown product of myelin, are elevated during SP EAE and MS (58). Since 15-HC activates microglial cells via a TLR2-PARP-1 axis, it could contribute to the extensive activation of microglia that characterises SPMS (58). Mitochondrial injury, the resulting energy crisis, and alterations in sodium channels are all thought to be important contributors to neurodegeneration and are potential therapeutic targets (reviewed in 57, 59).

The role of the adaptive immune system in MS
CD4+ T cells

Much of the research into MS and the animal model EAE have centred on CD4 T cells. The strongest genetic link for MS is with MHC class II genes. In the EAE model CD4 T cells have been strongly implicated in initiating disease since EAE can be induced by adoptive transfer of CD4 T cells specific for myelin antigens. Furthermore, knock-out mice have provided key information on the role of distinct cytokines in protection and pathology (Table 4.1).

Distinct subsets of CD4 T cells have been defined on the basis of their expression of cytokines and transcription factors. The differentiation of these CD4 T cell subsets from naïve T cells occurs when they are stimulated by their cognate antigen presented by an APC such as a DC (Figure 4.4) in the presence of polarizing cytokines. DCs produce regulatory cytokines in response to stimulation of one or more PRR by exogenous PAMPs or endogenous DAMPs, and these cytokines are crucial in determining the type of T helper cell response that ensues. IL-12 drives the differentiation of IFN-γ-producing Th1 cells, while IL-4 drives Th2 responses, characterised by production of IL-4, IL-5, and IL-13. More recently, Th17 cells have been described, and these differentiate under the influence

Table 4.1 The effect of manipulating T cell subsets and cytokines on the development of EAE

Molecule/ cell type [a]	Manipulation [b]	Background [c]	Induction method [d]	Effect on EAE [e]	Reference
IL-12p40	Genetic deletion	C57BL/6	MOG/CFA	**Resistant**	(60)
IL-12p35	Genetic deletion	C57BL/6	MOG/CFA	Susceptible	(60)
IL-23p19	Genetic deletion	B6x129	MOG/CFA	**Resistant**	(60, 61)
IL-6	Genetic deletion	129Sv × C57BL/6	MOG/CFA	**Resistant**	(62)
IL-1R	Genetic deletion	C57BL/6	MOG/CFA	**Resistant**	(63)
IFN-	Genetic deletion	B10.PL	MBP/CFA	Increased mortality Delayed resolution	(64)
IL-17	Genetic deletion	C57BL/6	MOG/CFA	Delayed onset Reduced severity	(65, 66[f])
IL-21/IL-21R	Genetic deletion	C57BL/6	MOG/CFA	Susceptible	(67)
IL-22	Genetic deletion	C57BL/6	MOG/CFA	Susceptible	(68)
IL-9/IL-9R	Neutralisation/ genetic deletion	C57BL/6	MOG/CFA	Delayed onset/ attenuated disease	(69)
GM-CSF	Genetic deletion	C57BL/6	MOG/CFA	**Resistant**	(70)
Th1	Adoptive transfer	C57BL/6	Th1 transfer	Induced disease	(71)
Th1	Adoptive transfer	SJL	Th1 transfer	Failed to induce disease	(72)
Th1	Adoptive transfer	SJL	Th1 transfer	Induced disease	(73)
Th17	Adoptive transfer	C57BL/6	Th17 transfer	Failed to induce disease	(71)
Th17	Adoptive transfer	SJL	Th17 transfer	Induced disease	(72, 73)

[a] Molecule or cell type of interest that was manipulated in each study.
[b] Approaches taken to manipulate cells or molecules include gene deletion, administration of neutralising antibody, or adoptive transfer of T cell lines.
[c] Mouse strain background.
[d] Methods used to induce EAE include active induction with myelin antigens plus CFA or passive induction by adoptive transfer of T cell lines.
[e] Effect of manipulation on the clinical symptoms of EAE.
[f] Found only marginal contribution after deletion of IL-17A and IL-17F.

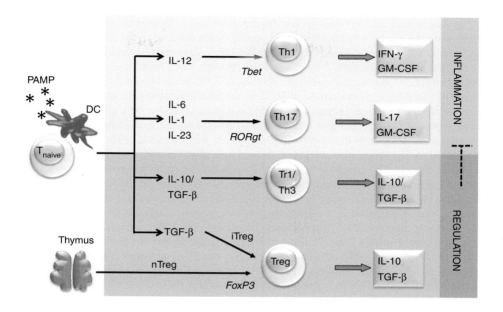

Figure 4.4. The development of CD4 T cells subsets involved in RRMS. Pathogenic Th1 and Th17 cells are thought to play a major role in the development of RRMS. Th1 cells differentiate from naïve cells that are primed in the presence of IL-12 and produce IFN-γ as their signature cytokine. Th17 cells differentiate under the influence of a combination of cytokines that can include IL-6, IL-1, IL-23, IL-21, and TGF-β. Th17 cells produce IL-17A, IL-17F, IL-9, and GM-CSF. Pathogenic autoreactive T cells are constrained by regulatory T cells which include Tr1 cells and nTreg cells. Tr1 and Th3 cells differentiate from naïve cells activated in the presence of IL-10 or TGF-β, respectively, and produce anti-inflammatory IL-10 or TGF-β. Fully differentiated nTreg cells emerge from the thymus and are thought to be specific for self antigens. iTreg cells, which are indistinguishable from nTreg cells, can also be generated in the periphery under the influence of TGF-β and retinoic acid.

of combinations of IL-1, IL-23, IL-6, IL-21, and TGF-β. Th17 cells produce IL-17A, IL-17F, granulocyte macrophage colony-stimulating factor (GM-CSF), IL-21, IL-9, IL-22, and TNF-α (60). Regulatory subsets of CD4 T cells include Tr1 cells which are driven by IL-10, induced Treg cells driven by TGF-β and retinoic acid, and natural Treg cells which emerge as fully differentiated cells directly from the thymus.

For many years Th1 cells were thought to be the key pathogenic T cells in EAE and MS. This was partly based on the observation that IL-12p40-defective (IL-12p40$^{-/-}$) mice were resistant to EAE, and IL-12 is required for differentiation of Th1 cells. In addition, treatment of MS patients with IFN-γ exacerbated disease (61). In contrast, however, IFN-γ$^{-/-}$ or STAT1$^{-/-}$ mice lacking Th1 cells developed more severe EAE (62, 63). The discovery of IL-23, which is structurally related to IL-12, partly resolved these paradoxes. IL-23 shares the p40 chain with IL-12, which associates with either a separate p19 or p35 chain to form IL-23 and IL-12, respectively. IL-23p19$^{-/-}$ mice, like the IL-12p40$^{-/-}$ mice, were found to be resistant to EAE; whereas IL-12p35$^{-/-}$ mice were susceptible (64), and IL-23 was essential to drive the induction or expansion of IL-17-secreting Th17 cells (65). Th17 cells have since been shown to promote inflammation and are pathogenic in many autoimmune disorders (60).

The central role of Th17 cells in the development and pathogenesis of EAE has been demonstrated in a number of studies. PLP-specific T cells cultured in the presence of IL-23 generated Th17 cell lines that induced EAE following passive transfer into naïve SJL mice, whereas Th1 cell lines generated by in vitro culture with IL-12 failed to induce EAE (65). Furthermore, IL-17 blockade reduced the severity of EAE, while blocking IFN-exacerbated disease (65). Similarly, neutralisation of IL-17 in the MOG-induced EAE model during the course of the disease modestly improved clinical symptoms (66). In one study IL-17$^{-/-}$ mice had very mild EAE, with delayed onset, reduced disease scores, and early recovery (67). However, in another study deletion of IL-17F together with blockade of IL-17A, which are both related to Th17 signature cytokines, showed only slight benefit (68). The disparity in the effects achieved by blocking IL-23, which resulted in complete resistance to EAE, versus the partial effect of blocking IL-17, suggested that other Th17-derived cytokines might also be involved, although IL-21 and IL-22 were found to be dispensable (69, 70). However, neutralisation of IL-9 attenuated EAE, suggesting a role for IL-9 in mediating Th17-mediated diseases (71). More recently, however, GM-CSF produced by Th17 cells has been shown to play a critical role in EAE (72, 73). IL-23 induces production of GM-CSF by Th17 cells (73). GM-CSF secretion by IFN-γ and IL-17-deficient T helper cells was sufficient to induce EAE, whereas T cells that expressed either IL-17 or IFN-γ in the absence of GM-CSF failed to initiate neuroinflammation (72). GM-CSF acted on infiltrating myeloid cells in the CNS to sustain neuroinflammation during the effector phase of EAE (72). Finally, GM-CSF-deficient mice represent the only Th17 cytokine knock-out to exhibit complete resistance to EAE (74) (Table 4.1).

Thus, although there has been some contradictory data on the relative importance of IL-17 and other Th17-derived cytokines in EAE, the consensus view that has emerged is that the Th17 cells have a clear pathogenic role in EAE and most likely in MS. Although early studies on Th17 cells dismissed a role for Th1 cells, recent data suggests that both cell types may play distinct roles in pathology. It has been reported that adoptive transfer of highly purified Th1 could induce EAE, whereas Th17 cells, devoid of IFN-γ-producing cells, could not induce disease (75). It was suggested that only Th1 cells could initially access the CNS, and that this facilitated subsequent recruitment of Th17 cells (75). T cells producing both IL-17 and IFN-γ, which express Tbet and RORγt, are also recruited to the CNS during EAE, and transferred Th17 cells can switch to IFN-γ production, indicating that there is plasticity within these populations (76, 77). It has also been suggested that the expression of Tbet defines the encephalogenicity of T cells rather than their cytokine profile (78), and inhibition of Tbet was shown to ameliorate EAE by inhibiting both Th1 and Th17 cells (79).

The vast data from the EAE model suggest that both Th1 and Th17 cells are likely to play a role in MS; however, the relative roles of Th1 and Th17 cells in MS and other human autoimmune diseases are still far from clear. Production of IL-17 and IFN-γ by T cells has been associated with disease activity in MS patients, and these cytokines are also expressed in brain lesions. Microarray analyses have detected IL-17 expression in MS brain lesions (80, 81), and enrichment of IL-17-producing cells, which included glial cells, CD4+, and CD8+ T cells, was identified in the active rather than inactive areas of MS brain lesions (82). Elevated frequencies of IL-17-producing cells have been associated with disease activity in the peripheral blood of MS patients (83, 84). However, it has also been reported that although IL-17 and IFN-γ were elevated very early in disease, only IFN-γ was associated with relapse (85). Human Th17 cells migrate more efficiently than Th1 cells in an in vitro BBB migration assay, and display cytotoxic activity against neurons (86). Interestingly, a recent study has identified an enrichment of T cells expressing both IL-17 and IFN-γ in MS brain tissue, suggesting that IL-17+IFN-γ+ T cells may be involved in pathology (87). On the basis of the data from the EAE model (72, 73), the potential role of Th17-derived GM-CSF will now need to be investigated in MS. However, elevated GM-CSF concentrations have been found during a cytokine screen of CSF from MS patients (88). GM-CSF is likely to play an important role in APC in the CNS, since it was shown that monocytes migrating across the inflamed human blood–brain barrier differentiated into DCs under the influence of TGF-β and GM-CSF, and these DCs promoted the differentiation of Th17 and Th1 cells (89).

A definite role for Th17 cells has been identified in patients with neuromyelitis optica (NMO), which selectively affects the optic nerve and spinal cord. In NMO there is a marked increase in the frequency of Th17 cells and concentration of serum IL-17, compared to both MS patients and controls (90, 91). Thus the pathogenesis of NMO involves not only aquaporin 4-specific antibody (discussed below), but also Th17 cells (92).

Clearly much of the focus in recent literature has been on the relative role of Th17 and Th1 cells in EAE and MS. However, while data from the EAE model has been very informative there is still much work to be done to understand the roles of these cells in MS. Studies in MS patients have provided evidence that Th1 and Th17 cells are active or expanded during disease, but their contribution to pathology has understandably been more difficult to define. Since MS is a heterogeneous disease, it is possible that future studies may define specific subtypes of MS associated with particular pathogenic cell types. For example, a recent study suggests that elevated expression of serum IL-7 in MS may be associated with Th1-driven disease (93); and the ability to define such subtypes of MS patients is likely to help predict the response to therapy (94).

CD8+ T cells

Although MS has historically been viewed as a CD4+ T cell-mediated autoimmune disease, in part due to the genetic association of MS with MHC class II alleles, more recently an association with MHC class I alleles has also been reported [95]. Furthermore, the frequency of CD8+ T cells is much greater than that of CD4+ T cells in inflammatory lesions, and CD8+ T cells show oligoclonal expansion in plaques, CSF, and blood, all suggestive of a pathogenic role in MS (96, 97). Myelin-reactive CD8 T cells have been identified at higher frequencies in MS compared with healthy controls (98), as have cytotoxic CD8 T cells expressing perforin (99). Although much of the focus has been on the role of Th17 cells, IL-17-secreting CD8 T cells were also recently shown to be increased in NMO and MS patients during relapse (91). Microarray studies performed in twins discordant for MS have identified disease-related differences in CD161 expression within the CD8 compartment (100). Furthermore, the frequency of CD8+CD161+IL-17+ cells was increased in MS patients, providing further evidence for a role of IL-17-producing CD8 T cells in MS (100). Analogous to CD4 T cells, CD8 T cells may play a dual role in MS, with regulatory as well as pathogenic functions (reviewed in (101)). Neuroantigen-specific regulatory CD8 T cells have been identified in MS patients and controls; however, they were dysfunctional in MS patients during relapse (102). Another study identified suppressive CD8+CD25+FoxP3+ cells, which were reduced in frequency in the blood and CSF of MS patients during relapse (103).

Cell transfer studies have suggested that CD8+ T cells are pathogenic in EAE (reviewed in (104)). However there is also evidence of a regulatory role for CD8+ T cells in EAE; EAE is more severe in mice deficient in or depleted of CD8+ T cells and disease severity has been inversely correlated with the frequency of CD8+ T cells (104). Furthermore, CD8+ Treg cells suppressed EAE via a TGF-β-dependent mechanism (105).

B cells

For many years there has been speculation about the possible role of B cells in MS, although clear evidence, such as that found in classical antibody-mediated autoimmune diseases such as myasthenia gravis, has been lacking. The presence of oligoclonal bands in the CSF is a classical diagnostic procedure for MS, suggesting that B cells undergo clonal expansion in the CNS during MS. Furthermore, B cells, plasma cells, and antibody are present in MS lesions. Until recently, however, there was little evidence regarding the pathogenicity or specificity of B cells in MS. In patients diagnosed with neuromyelitis optica (NMO), a variant of MS, a key role for B cells specific for aquaporin 4 has been identified (106, 107). Assays to detect the presence of specific aquaporin 4 antibodies in the serum have tested positive in the majority of NMO patients (108). Aquaporin 4-specific antibodies are strongly implicated in the pathogenesis of NMO, since there is a correlation between the levels of serum aquaporin 4-specific antibodies and disease activity (109, 110), and NMO-like disease can be transferred using aquaporin 4-specific antibody in animal models of disease (111, 112). Furthermore, in vitro studies have shown that aquaporin 4-positive serum has pathogenic effects (113). Autoantibodies specific for MOG have been detected in paediatric MS (12, 114).

The precise role and specificity of B cells in the more common forms of MS is less clear. However the success of rituximab treatment in MS clearly points to a pathogenic role for B cells in MS. Rituximab is a monoclonal antibody specific for CD20 on B cells, and treatment results in the lysis of B cells (115). In particular, rituximab has proved very effective in treating NMO (116, 117) and was accompanied by decreased aquaporin 4 antibody and memory B cells (116). Rituximab has also been effective in RRMS (115). The rapidity with which rituximab therapy takes effect in MS, without affecting antibody levels (118), suggests that B cell depletion may be effective through other mechanisms such as inhibiting antigen presentation by B cells or chemokine levels (119).

In summary, recent evidence suggests that B cells play an important pathogenic role in MS, and specific autoantibodies appear to play a pathogenic role in certain subgroups of patients. The success of rituximab treatment for MS also indicates a less obvious pathogenic role for B cells in MS, one that possibly is not mediated only via antibody but also via indirect effects of B cells upon other immune cells.

Regulatory T cells

Regulatory T (Treg) cells include both natural and adaptive Treg cells (Figure 4.4). Natural Treg (nTreg) cells express cell surface CD25 and the transcription factor FoxP3 which is essential for directing regulatory function (120, 121). nTreg cells were originally identified through their function in controlling autoimmunity by maintaining immunological toler-ance to self antigens (122). Fully differentiated nTreg cells are derived from the thymus, when CD4 T cells with higher than normal affinity for self antigens are positively selected, and such self antigen-specific nTreg cells are thought to play a dominant role in controlling autoreactive T cells (123). Treg cells that are indistinguishable from nTreg cells can also be induced in the periphery from naïve T cells activated in the presence of TGF-β and retinoic acid. Studies on human nTreg cells, particularly those in disease settings, can be compromised by the fact that many Treg cell markers including CD25 and FoxP3 may be up-regulated on activated effector cells. For this reason, $CD127^{lo}$ is now often used in addition to CD25 and FoxP3 to identify human nTreg cells (124).

Adaptive Treg cells, including Tr1, Th3, and various subsets of $CD8^+$ Treg cells, are derived in the periphery from uncommitted naïve T cells stimulated by antigen under the influence of the immunosuppressive cytokines IL-10 and TGF-β. Tr1 cells exert their suppressive function primarily via IL-10 secretion (125), whereas Th3 cells secrete high levels of TGF-β. Currently there are no specific markers to distinguish Tr1 and Th3 cells.

There is no doubt that the various types of Treg cells play a crucial role in maintaining immune homeostasis, and both natural and adaptive Treg cells are likely to regulate autoimmune inflammation during MS and EAE. Potentially autoreactive T cells specific for myelin antigens are present in healthy individuals, suggesting these cells are normally constrained by regulatory mechanisms which may be impaired in MS. Indeed, Tr1 responses have been shown to be reduced in MS patients, reflected in reduced levels of IL-10 (126, 127). While there have also been reports of reduced frequency of nTreg cells in MS patients (128), the majority of studies have found a similar frequency to that observed in normal individuals (129, 130). One study found a reduced frequency of nTreg cells in RRMS but not in SPMS (131), perhaps reflecting the fact that inflammation is thought to play a role in RRMS, but not in the progressive phase. Interestingly, an increased frequency of CD25+FoxP3+ nTreg cells has been found in the CSF but not the blood of MS patients (129).

Although there may be no numerical deficit in Treg cells in MS, studies using in vitro suppression assays have demonstrated that Treg cells from MS patients are functionally impaired (128–130, 132–138), which was reversed after therapy with IFN-β (137, 139), glatiramer acetate (140), or steroids (141). The discrepancy between the studies on Treg cells from MS patients may be due at least in part to the fact that Treg cell markers, such as CD25 and FoxP3, can be induced on effector T cells after activation and may therefore confound both phenotypic and functional studies in inflammatory settings. In the case of functional studies, sorting on the basis of $CD25^{hi}$ alone could have led to the inclusion of activated effector T cells, which would reduce the suppressive effect of the regulatory population. Indeed when $CD127^{lo}$ was used in addition to CD25 to sort Treg cells, there was no reduction in the suppressive function of Treg cells from MS patients compared with controls (142). The functional studies employed proliferation and/or production of IFN- as readouts for suppression of responder T cells, but did not examine the ability of Treg cells from MS patients to suppress IL-17 production by responder T cells. We have recently shown that a subset of Treg cells expressing CD39 were able to suppress both IFN and IL-17 in healthy controls; however, CD39+ Treg cells from RRMS patients had an impaired ability to suppress IL-17 (143), suggesting that there is defective regulation of IL-17 by nTreg cells from these patients. Treg subsets identified on the basis of HLA-DR expression were also recently shown to be functionally defective in MS patients (144). Since the majority of Treg cell studies in MS have been carried out in peripheral blood, it is unclear as to whether the data reflects the situation in the CNS. However, a recent histopathological study showed that Treg cells were low or absent within MS lesions, and those found within the CSF were highly apoptosis prone (145). A relative absence of Treg cells within MS lesions could be explained by the fact that Treg cells from MS patients exhibited reduced capacity to migrate across an endothelial barrier (146).

Adoptive transfer and depletion experiments in mice have provided definitive evidence that Treg can control the development and severity of EAE. In MOG-induced EAE, transfer of CD4+ CD25+ Treg cells reduced disease severity (147), and the protective effects were mediated by IL-10, since Treg cells from IL-10$^{-/-}$ mice failed to confer protection (148). In the PLP-induced model, the susceptibility of different mouse strains to EAE correlates inversely with the frequency of PLP-specific CD4+ CD25+ Treg cells (149). Furthermore, depletion of CD25+ cells rendered the resistant B10 mice susceptible to EAE (149) and increased susceptibility to suboptimally induced EAE (150). These studies suggest that Treg cells influence the susceptibility to and threshold of disease in the EAE models.

Immunomodulatory therapies for MS

All of the disease-modifying therapies (DMT) that are available for the treatment of MS have immunomodulatory effects on the immune system. Until recently, the number of treatment options for MS has been limited; however, new DMTs are now available which have improved efficacy, although this benefit has to be balanced against their side effect profiles. Biological therapies are also expensive, placing an increasing burden on health care systems. Furthermore, as discussed above the current therapeutic strategies are largely ineffective in PPMS and SPMS and therefore one of the major challenges ahead will be to develop effective therapies for use in the progressive forms of MS.

First-line therapy for RRMS

IFN-β has been in use for the treatment of RRMS since 1993. IFN-β is best known for its antiviral effects, and this was the rationale for its initial use in MS. Serendipitously, it proved to also have broad immunomodulatory effects which are of benefit in RRMS. There are three formulations of IFN-β available to treat MS; Betaseron is a non-glycosylated protein (IFN-β1b) produced in *E. coli*, while Avonex and Rebif are glycosylated forms of IFN-β (IFN-β1a) produced in CHO cells. These drugs are administered by injection from one to three times per week depending on the formulation, and some patients experience injection site side effects, flu-like symptoms, and depression. IFN-β has proved to be very safe in the long term; however, approximately half of those treated fail to respond to treatment. Non-responders are usually defined clinically as patients who experience more than one relapse per year, a sustained increase in EDSS, or new lesions on MRI while on treatment. The majority of treatment failure can be explained by the development of neutralising antibodies to IFN-β (151), the frequency of which varies according to the IFN-β formulation (152). However, other patients who fail IFN-β therapy in the absence of neutralising antibodies may have an inherent abnormality in the IFN-β signaling pathway.

Various different immunomodulatory effects have been ascribed to IFN-β, reflecting the pleiotropic nature of this cytokine. IFN-β helps to maintain the integrity of the BBB and has also been reported to skew the T cell cytokine response towards a less inflammatory profile. Recently IFN-β has been shown to inhibit the development and activity of Th17 cells (153), directly or via its effects on antigen-presenting cells such as dendritic cells, where it inhibited production of IL-1 and IL-23 and induced IL-27 (153). However, the role of Th17 cells in MS is still controversial. It has been suggested that disease may be either Th1 or Th17 mediated, and IFN-β therapy actually exacerbates Th17-mediated disease, which includes NMO (94, 97, 98).

Glatiramer acetate (GA) is the generic name for Copaxone®, which is a random polymer of four amino acids, designed to mimic myelin basic protein MBP. GA was developed in the EAE model where it was initially used with the aim of exacerbating disease; however, its unexpected immunomodulatory effect led to its development as a therapy for MS (154). GA is administered daily by injection, and has similar efficacy to IFN-β, reducing relapse rates by approximately one third (155). GA has a good side effect profile and has proven to be safe in the long term. Various broad immunomodulatory effects have been attributed to GA, including promiscuous binding to MHC class II molecules to prevent activation of autoantigen-specific T cells, skewing towards anti-inflammatory Th responses via modulation of cytokine production by APC, induction of regulatory responses including CD8 suppressor cells, regulatory CD4+ FoxP3+ T cells and regulatory B cells, and induction of neurotrophic factors (156).

Second-line therapies for RRMS

Natalizumab (Tysabri®) was the first MS drug developed with a targeted mechanism of action. It is a humanised antibody specific for the integrin VLA-4 (α4β1), which very effectively inhibits the ability of T cells to cross the BBB, and reduced the relapse rate by 68% (157). Natalizumab is administered by infusion once a month. After successful results in phase III trials, natalizumab was initially approved for the first-line treatment of RRMS, either alone or in combination with IFN-β. However, due to the development of progressive multifocal leukoencephalopathy (PML) in some patients, the drug is now only licensed for use in patients that have previously failed first-line therapy, or those with highly active disease (158). PML is a CNS infection with the JC virus, which is present as a persistent, asymptomatic infection in approximately 50–60% of the population. It is thought that natalizumab inhibits the normal surveillance of the CNS, allowing the JC virus to re-activate, causing potentially fatal neuroinflammation. The annualized risk of PML in patients who are seronegative for the JC virus is < 0.11 per 1000, which increases to between 0.35 and 8.1 per 1000 in seropositive patients, depending on the duration of treatment and history of previous immunosuppression (159). Thus current precautions include pre-treatment screening to determine prior infection with the JC virus, and patients who are JC virus positive are carefully monitored (160).

Fingolimod or FTY720 (Gilenya®) is the first oral therapy for MS; it was approved in 2010 by the US FDA for first-line treatment of RRMS and by the EMA in 2011 for second-line treatment of severe RRMS. This drug, which is a functional antagonist of the sphingosine-1-phosphate (S1P) receptor, was designed to target the trafficking of activated lymphocytes. Signaling via the S1P receptors on activated lymphocytes allows them to respond to a gradient of S1P concentration to leave the lymph nodes and traffic to the CNS; this is inhibited by fingolimod which binds to the receptors and causes their internalisation (161). Fingolimod appears to preferentially sequester naïve and CCR7$^+$ central memory T cells, while CCR7$^-$ effector memory T cells retain the ability to traffic (162). In addition, fingolimod has been suggested to have important direct effects on the CNS; it can enter the CNS and S1P receptors are expressed on neurons, astrocytes, and microglial cells (161). Potential beneficial effects of fingolimod in the CNS include improved survival of oligodendrocytes, myelin repair, and neuroprotective effects (161).

In phase III trials fingolimod reduced annual relapse rates compared to placebo or IFN-β (163, 164). Approximately 80% of patients on fingolimod therapy were relapse free compared with 69% on IFN-β (164). There are a number of potentially serious side effects associated with fingolimod. Bradycardia is a potential complication associated with the first oral dose of fingolimod in 1–3% of patients, requiring monitoring for 6 hours following the first administration (165). In addition, peripheral blood lymphocyte counts were severely reduced, liver enzymes elevated, and an increase in the incidence of skin cancers and infection was observed. Two deaths occurred during a phase III trial due to herpes virus infections, although corticosteroids were also administered to these patients (165). Thus screening measures prior to initiation of fingolimod treatment should include leucocyte counts, ECG, liver enzymes, and serum titres for herpes zoster virus; if seronegative then vaccination should be considered (165).

Emerging therapies

There are a number of other potential new therapies for MS which have shown benefit in clinical trials but are not yet approved for use in MS.

BG-12 (fumaric acid ester) is an oral drug that has previously been used for the treatment of psoriasis and more recently trialed for the treatment of RRMS. BG-12 has demonstrated superior efficacy to Copaxone and has a good side effect profile, which together with its oral administration make it an attractive option for a potential first-line therapy for RRMS. In two phase II trials BG-12 treatment reduced relapse rates by approximately 50% compared to placebo (166). The mechanism of action of BG-12 in MS is not well defined; however, its potential effects include neuroprotection via activation of nuclear factor E-related transcription factor which increases antioxidant protein expression (167). In addition it may exert anti-inflammatory effects by inhibiting NF-κB and modulating APC function (168).

Alemtuzumab (Campath) is a humanised monoclonal antibody specific for CD52, which depletes CD52-expressing immune cells including T cells, B cells, NK cells, and APC. Alemtuzumab is administered by an initial infusion, which is repeated after 1 year. The immune compartments gradually reconstitute although not usually back to baseline levels (169). In phase III trials alemtuzumab showed approximately a 50% reduction in relapse rate compared with IFN-β (166). Potential serious side effects include the development of secondary autoimmune disease (170).

Rituximab and the newer generation ocrelizumab are CD20-specific monoclonal antibodies which deplete B cells via antibody and complement-mediated lysis. The success of B cell depletion in MS has highlighted a previously unappreciated role for B cells in the pathogenesis of MS. In a phase II trial for ocrelizumab there was approximately a 90% reduction in new MRI lesions at 24 weeks compared with IFN-β (171). These data suggest that B cell depletion may be a promising strategy for MS; phase III trials are underway and these results will be required to establish safety and the longer term effect on disability.

Daclizumab is a monoclonal antibody specific for CD25 which is the α-subunit of the IL-2 receptor. The rationale for use of this drug was to deplete activated T cells which express CD25; however, it has been shown to also induce regulatory CD56^{bright} NK cells (30). In phase II trials the relapse rates were reduced from 0.46 for placebo to 0.21–0.23 for daclizumab. Phase III trials are underway and will help to confirm the efficacy and determine the safety profile of daclizumab.

Teriflunomide is an oral drug which is being considered for use in MS. Teriflunomide inhibits pyrimidine synthesis in rapidly dividing cells such as activated lymphocytes, thereby exerting immunomodulatory effects (166). In a phase II trial teriflunomide reduced relapses by approximately 30% compared with placebo and had no serious side effects (172); however, its potential teratogenic effects warrant caution.

Laquinomid is another oral drug under consideration for the treatment of MS. In animal models laquinomod was shown to exert anti-inflammatory effects on T cells via APC (173) and may also be neuroprotective (174). In phase III trials laquinimod showed approximately 23% reduction in relapse rate compared with placebo (175); however, the data suggest that its effect on disability progression may be more significant.

SPMS and PPMS

The DMTs used in RRMS are generally ineffective in SPMS and PPMS without relapse, and so the treatment options for patients with progressive MS are very limited. Mitoxantrone is an immuno-suppressive chemotherapeutic agent used for the treatment of SPMS, progressive–relapsing MS, or worsening RRMS. Mitoxantrone is administered every 3 months up to a maximum cumulative dose, and inhibits DNA synthesis and repair. Its mechanism of action includes reduction in CD4 T cell counts, inhibition of B cells, as well as effects on macrophages (176). The use of mitoxatrone is limited by serious side effects including cardiotoxicity and acute leukaemia.

Fampridine (Ampyra) is used to improve walking in MS patients, and improves nerve conductivity by inhibiting neuronal potassium channels (177).

Summary

Our understanding of the role of the immune system in MS has developed immensely over the past few years and has contributed to the development of more effective, targeted therapies. Early research into MS focused largely on the role of CD4 T cells, which are thought to be important in triggering MS. More recently, however, the importance of other components of the adaptive immune system such as B cells and CD8 T cells has been highlighted. These adaptive immune responses are shaped by innate responses and together these are thought to mediate the inflammation in the CNS during RRMS. Therapies that have anti-inflammatory or immunomodulatory effects are effective during RRMS; however, the more progressive forms of the disease are resistant to such treatment. Thus it appears that the disease processes involved in progressive disease differ from those in RRMS. Progressive MS is associated with neurodegenerative processes secondary to the inflammation during RRMS. There is increasing evidence of an important role for the innate immune system in perpetuating progressive disease.

References

1. Diaz-Villoslada, P., Shih, A., Shao, L., Genain, C.P., and Hauser, S.L. (1999). Autoreactivity to myelin antigens: myelin/oligodendrocyte glycoprotein is a prevalent autoantigen. *J. Neuroimmunol.* **99**, 36–43.

2. Kutzelnigg, A., Faber-Rod, J.C., Bauer, J., et al. (2007). Widespread demyelination in the cerebellar cortex in multiple sclerosis. *Brain Pathol.* **17**, 38–44.

3. Witte, M.E., Geurts, J.J., de Vries, H.E., van der Valk, P., and van Horssen, J. (2010). Mitochondrial dysfunction: a potential link between neuroinflammation and neurodegeneration? *Mitochondrion* **10**, 411–418.

4. Ota, K., Matsui, M., Milford, E.L., et al. (1990). T-cell recognition of an

immunodominant myelin basic protein epitope in multiple sclerosis. *Nature* **346**, 183–187.

5. Wucherpfennig, K.W., Zhang, J., Witek, C., *et al.* (1994). Clonal expansion and persistence of human T cells specific for an immunodominant myelin basic protein peptide. *J. Immunol.* **152**, 5581–5592.

6. Chou, Y.K., Henderikx, P., Vainiene, M., *et al.* (1991). Specificity of human T cell clones reactive to immunodominant epitopes of myelin basic protein. *J. Neurosci. Res.* **28**, 280–290.

7. Olsson, T., Zhi, W.W., Hojeberg, B., *et al.* (1990). Autoreactive T lymphocytes in multiple sclerosis determined by antigen-induced secretion of interferon-gamma. *J. Clin. Invest.* **86**, 981–985.

8. Tejada-Simon, M.V., Hong, J., Rivera, V.M., and Zhang, J.Z. (2001). Reactivity pattern and cytokine profile of T cells primed by myelin peptides in multiple sclerosis and healthy individuals. *Eur. J. Immunol.* **31**, 907–917.

9. Mazza, G., Ponsford, M., Lowrey, P., *et al.* (2002). Diversity and dynamics of the T-cell response to MBP in DR2+ve individuals. *Clin. Exp. Immunol.* **128**, 538–547.

10. Hong, J., Zang, Y.C., Li, S., Rivera, V.M., and Zhang, J.Z. (2004). Ex vivo detection of myelin basic protein-reactive T cells in multiple sclerosis and controls using specific TCR oligonucleotide probes. *Eur. J. Immunol.* **34**, 870–881.

11. Bielekova, B., Sung, M.H., Kadom, N., *et al.* (2004). Expansion and functional relevance of high-avidity myelin-specific CD4+ T cells in multiple sclerosis. *J. Immunol.* **172**, 3893–3904.

12. McLaughlin, K.A., Chitnis, T., Newcombe, J., *et al.* (2009). Age-dependent B cell autoimmunity to a myelin surface antigen in pediatric multiple sclerosis. *J. Immunol.* **183**, 4067–4076.

13. McMahon, E.J., Bailey, S.L., Castenada, C.V., Waldner, H., and Miller, S.D. (2005). Epitope spreading initiates in the CNS in two mouse models of multiple sclerosis. *Nat. Med.* **11**, 335–339.

14. Klehmet, J., Shive, C., Guardia-Wolff, R., *et al.* (2004). T cell epitope spreading to myelin oligodendrocyte glycoprotein in HLA-DR4 transgenic mice during experimental autoimmune encephalomyelitis. *Clin. Immunol.* **111**, 53–60.

15. Davies, S., Nicholson, T., Laura, M., Giovannoni, G., and Altmann, D.M. (2005). Spread of T lymphocyte immune responses to myelin epitopes with duration of multiple sclerosis. *J. Neuropathol. Exp. Neurol.* **64**, 371–377.

16. Kutzelnigg, A., Lucchinetti, C.F., Stadelmann, C., *et al.* (2005). Cortical demyelination and diffuse white matter injury in multiple sclerosis. *Brain* **128**, 2705–2712.

17. Weiner, H.L. (2009). The challenge of multiple sclerosis: how do we cure a chronic heterogeneous disease? *Ann. Neurol.* **65**, 239–248.

18. Bailey-Bucktrout, S.L., Caulkins, S.C., Goings, G., *et al.* (2008). Cutting edge: central nervous system plasmacytoid dendritic cells regulate the severity of relapsing experimental autoimmune encephalomyelitis. *J. Immunol.* **180**, 6457–6461.

19. Bailey, S.L., Schreiner, B., McMahon, E.J., and Miller, S.D. (2007). CNS myeloid DCs presenting endogenous myelin peptides 'preferentially' polarize CD4+ T(H)-17 cells in relapsing EAE. *Nat. Immunol.* **8**, 172–180.

20. Vaknin-Dembinsky, A., Balashov, K., and Weiner, H.L. (2006). IL-23 is increased in dendritic cells in multiple sclerosis and down-regulation of IL-23 by antisense oligos increases dendritic cell IL-10 production. *J. Immunol.* **176**, 7768–7774.

21. Karni, A., Abraham, M., Monsonego, A., *et al.* (2006). Innate immunity in multiple sclerosis: myeloid dendritic cells in secondary progressive multiple sclerosis are activated and drive a proinflammatory immune response. *J. Immunol.* **177**, 4196–4202.

22. Stasiolek, M., Bayas, A., Kruse, N., *et al.* (2006). Impaired maturation and altered regulatory function of plasmacytoid dendritic cells in multiple sclerosis. *Brain* **129**, 1293–1305.

23. Ajami, B., Bennett, J.L., Krieger, C., McNagny, K.M., and Rossi, F.M.

Infiltrating monocytes trigger EAE progression, but do not contribute to the resident microglia pool. *Nat. Neurosci.* **14**, 1142–1149.

24. Benveniste, E.N. (1997). Role of macrophages/microglia in multiple sclerosis and experimental allergic encephalomyelitis. *J. Mol. Med. (Berl.)* **75**, 165–173.

25. Traugott, U. (1985). Characterization and distribution of lymphocyte subpopulations in multiple sclerosis plaques versus autoimmune demyelinating lesions. *Springer Semin. Immunopathol.* **8**, 71–95.

26. Cooper, M.A., Fehniger, T.A., and Caligiuri, M.A. (2001). The biology of human natural killer-cell subsets. *Trends Immunol.* **22**, 633–640.

27. Pandya, A.D., Al-Jaderi, Z., Hoglund, R.A., *et al.* (2011). Identification of human NK17/NK1 cells. *PLoS One* **6**, e26780.

28. Hao, J., Liu, R., Piao, W., *et al.* (2010). Central nervous system (CNS)-resident natural killer cells suppress Th17 responses and CNS autoimmune pathology. *J. Exp. Med.* **207**, 1907–1921.

29. De Jager, P.L., Rossin, E., Pyne, S., *et al.* (2008). Cytometric profiling in multiple sclerosis uncovers patient population structure and a reduction of CD8low cells. *Brain* **131**, 1701–1711.

30. Bielekova, B., Catalfamo, M., Reichert-Scrivner, S., *et al.* (2006). Regulatory CD56 (bright) natural killer cells mediate immunomodulatory effects of IL-2R alpha-targeted therapy (daclizumab) in multiple sclerosis. *Proc. Natl. Acad. Sci. U. S. A.* **103**, 5941–5946.

31. Martinez-Rodriguez, J.E., Saez-Borderias, A., Munteis, E., *et al.* (2011). Natural killer receptors distribution in multiple sclerosis: relation to clinical course and interferon-beta therapy. *Clin. Immunol.* **137**, 41–50.

32. Berzins, S.P., Smyth, M.J., and Baxter, A.G. (2011). Presumed guilty: natural killer T cell defects and human disease. *Nat. Rev. Immunol.* **11**, 131–142.

33. Gigli, G., Caielli, S., Cutuli, D., and Falcone, M. (2007). Innate immunity modulates autoimmunity: type 1 interferon-beta treatment in multiple sclerosis promotes growth and function of regulatory invariant natural killer T cells through dendritic cell maturation. *Immunology* **122**, 409–417.

34. Wucherpfennig, K.W., Newcombe, J., Li, H., *et al.* (1992). Gamma delta T-cell receptor repertoire in acute multiple sclerosis lesions. *Proc. Natl. Acad. Sci. U. S. A.* **89**, 4588–4592.

35. Shimonkevitz, R., Colburn, C., Burnham, J.A., *et al.* (1993). Clonal expansions of activated gamma/delta T cells in recent-onset multiple sclerosis. *Proc. Natl. Acad. Sci. U. S. A.* **90**, 923–927.

36. Rajan, A.J., Gao, Y.L., Raine, C.S., and Brosnan, C.F. (1996). A pathogenic role for gamma delta T cells in relapsing-remitting experimental allergic encephalomyelitis in the SJL mouse. *J. Immunol.* **157**, 941–949.

37. Rajan, A.J., Klein, J.D., and Brosnan, C.F. (1998). The effect of gamma delta T cell depletion on cytokine gene expression in experimental allergic encephalomyelitis. *J. Immunol.* **160**, 5955–5962.

38. Spahn, T.W., Issazadah, S., Salvin, A.J., and Weiner, H.L. (1999). Decreased severity of myelin oligodendrocyte glycoprotein peptide 33–35-induced experimental autoimmune encephalomyelitis in mice with a disrupted TCR delta chain gene. *Eur. J. Immunol.* **29**, 4060–4071.

39. Odyniec, A., Szczepanik, M., Mycko, M.P., Stasiolek, M., Raine, C.S., and Selmaj, K.W. (2004). Gamma delta T cells enhance the expression of experimental autoimmune encephalomyelitis by promoting antigen presentation and IL-12 production. *J. Immunol.* **173**, 682–694.

40. Cardona, A.E. and Teale, J.M. (2002). Gamma/delta T cell-deficient mice exhibit reduced disease severity and decreased inflammatory response in the brain in murine neurocysticercosis. *J. Immunol.* **169**, 3163–3171.

41. Kobayashi, Y., Kawai, K., Ito, K., Honda, H., Sobue, G., and Yoshikai, Y. (1997). Aggravation of murine experimental allergic encephalomyelitis by administration of T-cell receptor gamma delta-specific antibody. *J. Neuroimmunol.* **73**, 169–174.

42. Ponomarev, E.D. and Dittel, B.N. (2005). Gamma delta T cells regulate the extent and duration of inflammation in the central nervous system by a Fas ligand-dependent mechanism. *J. Immunol.* **174**, 4678–4687.

43. Ponomarev, E.D., Novikova, M., Yassai, M., Szczepanik, M., Gorski, J., and Dittel, B.N. (2004). Gamma delta T cell regulation of IFN-gamma production by central nervous system-infiltrating encephalitogenic T cells: correlation with recovery from experimental autoimmune encephalomyelitis. *J. Immunol.* **173**, 1587–1595.

44. Lockhart, E., Green, A.M., and Flynn, J.L. (2006). IL-17 production is dominated by gamma delta T cells rather than CD4 T cells during *Mycobacterium tuberculosis* infection. *J. Immunol.* **177**, 4662–4669.

45. Shibata, K., Yamada, H., Hara, H., Kishihara, K., and Yoshikai, Y. (2007). Resident Vdelta1+ gamma delta T cells control early infiltration of neutrophils after *Escherichia coli* infection via IL-17 production. *J. Immunol.* **178**, 4466–4472.

46. Sutton, C.E., Lalor, S.J., Sweeney, C.M., Brereton, C.F., Lavelle, E.C., and Mills, K.H. (2009). Interleukin-1 and IL-23 induce innate IL-17 production from gamma delta T cells, amplifying Th17 responses and autoimmunity. *Immunity* **31**, 331–341.

47. Stinissen, P., Vandevyver, C., Medaer, R., et al. (1995). Increased frequency of gamma delta T cells in cerebrospinal fluid and peripheral blood of patients with multiple sclerosis: reactivity, cytotoxicity, and T cell receptor V gene rearrangements. *J. Immunol.* **154**, 4883–4894.

48. Chen, Z. and Freedman, M.S. (2008). Correlation of specialized CD16(+) gamma delta T cells with disease course and severity in multiple sclerosis. *J. Neuroimmunol.* **194**, 147–152.

49. Freedman, M.S., Ruijs, T.C., Selin, L.K., and Antel, J.P. (1991). Peripheral blood gamma-delta T cells lyse fresh human brain-derived oligodendrocytes. *Ann. Neurol.* **30**, 794–800.

50. Prinz, M., Garbe, F., Schmidt, H., et al. (2006). Innate immunity mediated by TLR9 modulates pathogenicity in an animal model of multiple sclerosis. *J. Clin. Invest.* **116**, 456–464.

51. Berer, K., Mues, M., Koutrolos, M. (2011). Commensal microbiota and myelin autoantigen cooperate to trigger autoimmune demyelination. *Nature* **479**, 538–541.

52. Bsibsi, M., Ravid, R., Gveric, D., and van Noort, J.M. (2002). Broad expression of Toll-like receptors in the human central nervous system. *J. Neuropathol. Exp. Neurol.* **61**, 1013–1021.

53. Correale, J., Fiol, M., and Gilmore, W. (2006). The risk of relapses in multiple sclerosis during systemic infections. *Neurology* **67**, 652–659.

54. Andersson, A., Covacu, R., Sunnemark, D., et al. (2008). Pivotal advance: HMGB1 expression in active lesions of human and experimental multiple sclerosis. *J. Leukoc. Biol.* **84**, 1248–1255.

55. Touil, T., Fitzgerald, D., Zhang, G.X., Rostami, A., and Gran, B. (2006). Cutting edge: TLR3 stimulation suppresses experimental autoimmune encephalomyelitis by inducing endogenous IFN-beta. *J. Immunol.* **177**, 7505–7509.

56. Gandhi, R., Laroni, A., and Weiner, H.L. (2010). Role of the innate immune system in the pathogenesis of multiple sclerosis. *J. Neuroimmunol.* **221**, 7–14.

57. van Horssen, J., Witte, M.E., Schreibelt, G., and de Vries, H.E. (2011). Radical changes in multiple sclerosis pathogenesis. *Biochim. Biophys. Acta* **1812**, 141–150.

58. Farez, M.F., Quintana, F.J., Gandhi, R., Izquierdo, G., Lucas, M., and Weiner, H.L. (2009). Toll-like receptor 2 and poly (ADP-ribose) polymerase 1 promote central nervous system neuroinflammation in progressive EAE. *Nat. Immunol.* **10**, 958–964.

59. Lassmann, H. and van Horssen, J. (2011). The molecular basis of neurodegeneration

in multiple sclerosis. *FEBS Lett.* **585**, 3715–3723.

60. Cua, D.J., Sherlock, J., Chen, Y., *et al.* (2003). Interleukin-23 rather than interleukin-12 is the critical cytokine for autoimmune inflammation of the brain. *Nature* **421**, 744–748.

61. Thakker, P., Leach, M.W., Kuang, W., Benoit, S.E., Leonard, J.P., and Marusic, S. (2007). IL-23 is critical in the induction but not in the effector phase of experimental autoimmune encephalomyelitis. *J. Immunol.* **178**, 2589–2598.

62. Eugster, H.P., Frei, K., Kopf, M., Lassmann, H., and Fontana, A. (1998). IL-6-deficient mice resist myelin oligodendrocyte glycoprotein-induced autoimmune encephalomyelitis. *Eur. J. Immunol.* **28**, 2178–2187.

63. Sutton, C., Brereton, C., Keogh, B., Mills, K.H., and Lavelle, E.C. (2006). A crucial role for interleukin (IL)-1 in the induction of IL-17-producing T cells that mediate autoimmune encephalomyelitis. *J. Exp. Med.* **203**, 1685–1691.

64. Ferber, I.A., Brocke, S., Taylor-Edwards, C., *et al.* (1996). Mice with a disrupted IFN-gamma gene are susceptible to the induction of experimental autoimmune encephalomyelitis (EAE). *J. Immunol.* **156**, 5–7.

65. Komiyama, Y., Nakae, S., Matsuki T., *et al.* (2006). IL-17 plays an important role in the development of experimental autoimmune encephalomyelitis. *J. Immunol.* **177**, 566–573.

66. Haak, S., Croxford, A.L., Kreymborg, K., *et al.* (2009). IL-17A and IL-17F do not contribute vitally to autoimmune neuro-inflammation in mice. *J. Clin. Invest.* **119**, 61–69.

67. Coquet, J.M., Chakravarti, S., Smyth, M.J., and Godfrey, D.I. (2008). Cutting edge: IL-21 is not essential for Th17 differentiation or experimental autoimmune encephalomyelitis. *J. Immunol.* **180**, 7097–7101.

68. Kreymborg, K., Etzensperger, R., Dumoutier, L., *et al.* (2007). IL-22 is expressed by Th17 cells in an IL-23-dependent fashion, but not required for the development of autoimmune encephalomyelitis. *J. Immunol.* **179**, 8098–8104.

69. Nowak, E.C., Weaver, C.T., Turner, H., *et al.* (2009). IL-9 as a mediator of Th17-driven inflammatory disease. *J. Exp. Med.* **206**, 1653–1660.

70. McQualter, J.L., Darwiche, R., Ewing, C., *et al.* (2001). Granulocyte macrophage colony-stimulating factor: a new putative therapeutic target in multiple sclerosis. *J. Exp. Med.* **194**, 873–882.

71. O'Connor, R.A., Prendergast, C.T., Sabatos, C.A., *et al.* (2008). Cutting edge: Th1 cells facilitate the entry of Th17 cells to the central nervous system during experimental autoimmune encephalomyelitis. *J. Immunol.* **181**, 3750–3754.

72. Langrish, C.L., Chen, Y., Blumenschein, W.M., *et al.* (2005). IL-23 drives a pathogenic T cell population that induces autoimmune inflammation. *J. Exp. Med.* **201**, 233–240.

73. Kroenke, M.A., Carlson, T.J., Andjelkovic, A.V., and Segal, B.M. (2008). IL-12- and IL-23-modulated T cells induce distinct types of EAE based on histology, CNS chemokine profile, and response to cytokine inhibition. *J. Exp. Med.* **205**, 1535–1541.

74. Harrington, L.E., Hatton, R.D., Mangan, P.R., *et al.* (2005). Interleukin 17-producing CD4+ effector T cells develop via a lineage distinct from the T helper type 1 and 2 lineages. *Nat. Immunol.* **6**, 1123–1132.

75. Panitch, H.S., Hirsch, R.L., and Haley, A.S., Johnson, K.P. (1987). Exacerbations of multiple sclerosis in patients treated with gamma interferon. *Lancet* **1**, 893–895.

76. Bettelli, E., Sullivan, B., Szabo, S.J., Sobel, R.A., Glimcher, L.H., and Kuchroo, V.K. (2004). Loss of T-bet, but not STAT1, prevents the development of experimental autoimmune encephalomyelitis. *J. Exp. Med.* **200**, 79–87.

77. Hofstetter, H.H., Ibrahim, S.M., Koczan, D., *et al.* (2005). Therapeutic efficacy of IL-17 neutralization in murine experimental autoimmune encephalomyelitis. *Cell Immunol.* **237**, 123–130.

78. Codarri, L., Gyulveszi, G., Tosevski, V., et al. (2011). RORgammat drives production of the cytokine GM-CSF in helper T cells, which is essential for the effector phase of autoimmune neuroinflammation. *Nat. Immunol.* **12**, 560–567.

79. El-Behi, M., Ciric, B., Dai, H., et al. (2011). The encephalitogenicity of T(H)17 cells is dependent on IL-1- and IL-23-induced production of the cytokine GM-CSF. *Nat. Immunol.* **12**, 568–575.

80. Abromson-Leeman, S., Bronson, R.T., and Dorf, M.E. (2009). Encephalitogenic T cells that stably express both T-bet and RORgammat consistently produce IFNgamma but have a spectrum of IL-17 profiles. *J Neuroimmunol.* **215**, 10–24.

81. Shi, G., Cox, C.A., Vistica, B.P., Tan, C., Wawrousek, E.F., and Gery, I. (2008). Phenotype switching by inflammation-inducing polarized Th17 cells, but not by Th1 cells. *J. Immunol.* **181**, 7205–7213.

82. Yang, Y., Weiner, J., Liu, Y., et al. (2009). T-bet is essential for encephalitogenicity of both Th1 and Th17 cells. *J. Exp. Med.* **206**, 1549–1564.

83. Gocke, A.R., Cravens, P.D., Ben, L.H., et al. (2007). T-bet regulates the fate of Th1 and Th17 lymphocytes in autoimmunity. *J. Immunol.* **178**, 1341–1348.

84. Lock, C., Hermans, G., Pedotti, R., et al. (2002). Gene-microarray analysis of multiple sclerosis lesions yields new targets validated in autoimmune encephalomyelitis. *Nat. Med.* **8**, 500–508.

85. Montes, M., Zhang, X., Berthelot, L., et al. (2009). Oligoclonal myelin-reactive T-cell infiltrates derived from multiple sclerosis lesions are enriched in Th17 cells. *Clin. Immunol.* **130**, 133–144.

86. Tzartos, J.S., Friese, M.A., Craner, M.J., et al. (2008). Interleukin-17 production in central nervous system-infiltrating T cells and glial cells is associated with active disease in multiple sclerosis. *Am. J. Pathol.* **172**, 146–155.

87. Matusevicius, D., Kivisakk, P., He, B., et al. (1999). Interleukin-17 mRNA expression in blood and CSF mononuclear cells is augmented in multiple sclerosis. *Mult. Scler.* **5**, 101–104.

88. Durelli, L., Conti, L., Clerico, M., et al. (2009). T-helper 17 cells expand in multiple sclerosis and are inhibited by interferon-beta. *Ann. Neurol.* **65**, 499–509.

89. Frisullo, G., Nociti, V., Iorio, R., et al. (2008). IL17 and IFNgamma production by peripheral blood mononuclear cells from clinically isolated syndrome to secondary progressive multiple sclerosis. *Cytokine* **44**, 22–25.

90. Kebir, H., Kreymborg, K., Ifergan, I., et al. (2007). Human TH17 lymphocytes promote blood-brain barrier disruption and central nervous system inflammation. *Nat. Med.* **13**, 1173–1175.

91. Kebir, H., Ifergan, I., Alvarez, J.I., et al. (2009). Preferential recruitment of interferon-gamma-expressing T(H)17 cells in multiple sclerosis. *Ann. Neurol.* **66**, 390–402.

92. Uzawa, A., Mori, M., Arai, K., et al. (yr). Cytokine and chemokine profiles in neuromyelitis optica: significance of interleukin-6. *Mult. Scler.* **16**, 1443–1452.

93. Ifergan, I., Kebir, H., Bernard, M., et al. (2008). The blood-brain barrier induces differentiation of migrating monocytes into Th17-polarizing dendritic cells. *Brain* **131**, 785–799.

94. Li, Y., Wang, H., Long, Y., Lu, Z., and Hu, X. (2011). Increased memory Th17 cells in patients with neuromyelitis optica and multiple sclerosis. *J. Neuroimmunol.* **234**, 155–160.

95. Wang, H.H., Dai, Y.Q., Qiu, W., et al. (2011). Interleukin-17-secreting T cells in neuromyelitis optica and multiple sclerosis during relapse. *J. Clin. Neurosci.* **18**, 1313–1317.

96. Kira, J. (2011). Neuromyelitis optica and opticospinal multiple sclerosis: mechanisms and pathogenesis. *Pathophysiology* **18**, 69–79.

97. Lee, L.F., Axtell, R., Tu, G.H., et al. (2011). IL-7 promotes T(H)1 development and serum IL-7 predicts clinical response to interferon-beta in multiple sclerosis. *Sci. Transl. Med.* **3**, 93ra68.

98. Axtell, R.C., Raman, C., and Steinman, L. (2011). Interferon-beta exacerbates Th17-mediated inflammatory disease. *Trends Immunol.* **32**, 272–277.

99. Sawcer, S., Ban, M., Maranian, M., *et al.* (2005). A high-density screen for linkage in multiple sclerosis. *Am. J. Hum.Genet.* **77**, 454–467.

100. Friese, M.A. and Fugger, L. (2009). Pathogenic CD8(+) T cells in multiple sclerosis. *Ann. Neurol.* **66**, 132–141.

101. Biegler, B.W., Yan, S.X., Ortega, S.B., Tennakoon, D.K., Racke, M.K., and Karandikar, N.J. (2011). Clonal composition of neuroantigen-specific CD8+ and CD4+ T-cells in multiple sclerosis. *J. Neuroimmunol.* **234**, 131–140.

102. Crawford, M.P., Yan, S.X., Ortega, S.B., *et al.* (2004). High prevalence of autoreactive, neuroantigen-specific CD8+ T cells in multiple sclerosis revealed by novel flow cytometric assay. *Blood* **103**, 4222–4231.

103. Giovanni, F., Domenico, P., Alessandro, M., *et al.* (2011). Circulating CD8(+) CD56(-)perforin(+) T cells are increased in multiple sclerosis patients. *J. Neuroimmunol.* **240–241**, 137–141.

104. Annibali, V., Ristori, G., Angelini, D.F., *et al.* (2011). CD161(high)CD8+T cells bear pathogenetic potential in multiple sclerosis. *Brain* **134**, 542–554.

105. Saxena, A., Martin-Blondel, G., Mars, L.T., and Liblau, R.S. (2011). Role of CD8 T cell subsets in the pathogenesis of multiple sclerosis. *FEBS Lett.* **585**, 3758–3763.

106. Baughman, E.J., Mendoza, J.P., Ortega, S.B., *et al.* (2011). Neuroantigen-specific CD8+ regulatory T-cell function is deficient during acute exacerbation of multiple sclerosis. *J. Autoimmun.* **36**, 115–124.

107. Correale, J. and Villa, A. (2010). Role of CD8+ CD25+ Foxp3+ regulatory T cells in multiple sclerosis. *Ann. Neurol.* **67**, 625–638.

108. Weiss, H.A., Millward, J.M., and Owens, T. (2007). CD8+ T cells in inflammatory demyelinating disease. *J. Neuroimmunol.* **191**, 79–85.

109. Chen, M.L., Yan, B.S., Kozoriz, D., and Weiner, H.L. (2009). Novel CD8(+) regulatory T cells suppress experimental autoimmune encephalomyelitis by TGF-beta- and IFN-gamma-dependent mechanisms. *Eur. J. Immunol.* **39**, 3423–3435.

110. Lennon, V.A., Kryzer, T.J., Pittock, S.J., Verkman, A.S., and Hinson, S.R. (2005). IgG marker of optic-spinal multiple sclerosis binds to the aquaporin-4 water channel. *J. Exp. Med.* **202**, 473–477.

111. Roemer, S.F., Parisi, J.E., Lennon, V.A., *et al.* (2007). Pattern-specific loss of aquaporin-4 immunoreactivity distinguishes neuromyelitis optica from multiple sclerosis. *Brain* **130**, 1194–1205.

112. Jarius, S., Probst, C., Borowski, K., *et al.* (2010). Standardized method for the detection of antibodies to aquaporin-4 based on a highly sensitive immunofluorescence assay employing recombinant target antigen. *J. Neurol. Sci.* **291**, 52–56.

113. Takahashi, T., Fujihara, K., Nakashima, I., *et al.* (2007). Anti-aquaporin-4 antibody is involved in the pathogenesis of NMO: a study on antibody titre. *Brain* **130**, 1235–1243.

114. Jarius, S., Aboul-Enein, F., Waters, P., *et al.* (2008). Antibody to aquaporin-4 in the long-term course of neuromyelitis optica. *Brain* **131**, 3072–3080.

115. Kinoshita, M., Nakatsuji, Y., Kimura, T., *et al.* (2009). Neuromyelitis optica: passive transfer to rats by human immunoglobulin. *Biochem. Biophys. Res. Commun.* **386**, 623–627.

116. Bradl, M., Misu, T., Takahashi, T., *et al.* (2009). Neuromyelitis optica: pathogenicity of patient immunoglobulin in vivo. *Ann. Neurol.* **66**, 630–643.

117. Hinson, S.R., Pittock, S.J., Lucchinetti, C.F., *et al.* (2007). Pathogenic potential of IgG binding to water channel extracellular domain in neuromyelitis optica. *Neurology* **69**, 2221–2231.

118. Probstel, A.K., Dornmair, K., Bittner, R., *et al.* (2011). Antibodies to MOG are

transient in childhood acute disseminated encephalomyelitis. *Neurology* 77, 580–588.

119. Hauser, S.L., Waubant, E., Arnold, D.L., et al. (2008). B-cell depletion with rituximab in relapsing-remitting multiple sclerosis. *N. Engl. J. Med.* 358, 676–688.

120. Kim, S.H., Kim, W., Li, X.F., Jung, I.J., and Kim, H.J. (2011). Repeated treatment with rituximab based on the assessment of peripheral circulating memory B cells in patients with relapsing neuromyelitis optica over 2 years. *Arch. Neurol.* 68, 1412–1420.

121. Bedi, G.S., Brown, A.D., Delgado, S.R., Usmani, N., Lam, B.L., and Sheremata, W.A. (2011). Impact of rituximab on relapse rate and disability in neuromyelitis optica. *Mult. Scler.* 17, 1225–1230.

122. Petereit, H.F., Moeller-Hartmann, W., Reske, D., and Rubbert, A. (2008). Rituximab in a patient with multiple sclerosis: effect on B cells, plasma cells and intrathecal IgG synthesis. *Acta. Neurol. Scand.* 117, 399–403.

123. Piccio, L., Naismith, R.T., Trinkaus, K., et al. (2010). Changes in B- and T-lymphocyte and chemokine levels with rituximab treatment in multiple sclerosis. *Arch. Neurol.* 67, 707–714.

124. Hori, S., and Sakaguchi, S. (2004). Foxp3: a critical regulator of the development and function of regulatory T cells. *Microbes Infect.* 6, 745–751.

125. Fontenot, J.D., Gavin, M.A., and Rudensky, A.Y. (2003). Foxp3 programs the development and function of CD4+CD25+ regulatory T cells. *Nat. Immunol.* 4, 330–336.

126. Sakaguchi, S., Sakaguchi, N., Asano, M., Itoh, M., and Toda, M. (1995). Immunologic self-tolerance maintained by activated T cells expressing IL-2 receptor alpha-chains (CD25): breakdown of a single mechanism of self-tolerance causes various autoimmune diseases. *J. Immunol.* 155, 1151–1164.

127. Liston, A. and Rudensky, A.Y. (2007). Thymic development and peripheral homeostasis of regulatory T cells. *Curr. Opin. Immunol.* 19, 176–185.

128. Liu, W., Putnam, A.L., Xu-Yu, Z., et al. (2006). CD127 expression inversely correlates with FoxP3 and suppressive function of human CD4+ T reg cells. *J. Exp. Med.* 203, 1701–1711.

129. Roncarolo, M.G., Gregori, S., Battaglia, M., Bacchetta, R., Fleischhauer, K., and Levings, M.K. (2006). Interleukin-10-secreting type 1 regulatory T cells in rodents and humans. *Immunol. Rev.* 212, 28–50.

130. Martinez-Forero, I., Garcia-Munoz, R., Martinez-Pasamar, S., et al. (2008). IL-10 suppressor activity and ex vivo Tr1 cell function are impaired in multiple sclerosis. *Eur. J. Immunol.* 38, 576–586.

131. Astier, A.L., Meiffren, G., Freeman, S., and Hafler, D.A. (2006). Alterations in CD46-mediated Tr1 regulatory T cells in patients with multiple sclerosis. *J. Clin. Invest.* 116, 3252–3257.

132. Venken, K., Hellings, N., Thewissen, M., et al. (2008). Compromised CD4+ CD25 (high) regulatory T-cell function in patients with relapsing-remitting multiple sclerosis is correlated with a reduced frequency of FOXP3-positive cells and reduced FOXP3 expression at the single-cell level. *Immunology* 123, 79–89.

133. Feger, U., Luther, C., Poeschel, S., Melms, A., Tolosa, E., and Wiendl, H., et al. (2007). Increased frequency of CD4+ CD25+ regulatory T cells in the cerebrospinal fluid but not in the blood of multiple sclerosis patients. *Clin. Exp. Immunol.* 147, 412–418.

134. Haas, J., Hug, A., Viehover, A., et al. (2005). Reduced suppressive effect of CD4+CD25high regulatory T cells on the T cell immune response against myelin oligodendrocyte glycoprotein in patients with multiple sclerosis. *Eur. J. Immunol.* 35, 3343–3352.

135. Venken, K., Hellings, N., Hensen, K., et al. (2006). Secondary progressive in contrast to relapsing-remitting multiple sclerosis patients show a normal CD4+CD25+ regulatory T-cell function

and FOXP3 expression. *J. Neurosci. Res.* **83**, 1432–1446.

136. Viglietta, V., Baecher-Allan, C., Weiner, H.L., and Hafler, D.A. (2004). Loss of functional suppression by CD4+CD25+ regulatory T cells in patients with multiple sclerosis. *J. Exp. Med.* **199**, 971–979.

137. Tsaknaridis, L., Spencer, L., Culbertson, N., *et al.* (2003). Functional assay for human CD4+CD25+ Treg cells reveals an age-dependent loss of suppressive activity. *J. Neurosci. Res.* **74**, 296–308.

138. Huan, J., Culbertson, N., Spencer, L., *et al.* (2005). Decreased FOXP3 levels in multiple sclerosis patients. *J. Neurosci. Res.* **81**, 45–52.

139. Frisullo, G., Nociti, V., Iorio, R., *et al.* (2008). Regulatory T cells fail to suppress CD4(+)T-bet(+) T cells in relapsing multiple sclerosis patients. *Immunology* **127**, 418–428.

140. Venken, K., Thewissen, M., Hellings, N., *et al.* (2007). A CFSE based assay for measuring CD4+CD25+ regulatory T cell mediated suppression of auto-antigen specific and polyclonal T cell responses. *J. Immunol. Methods.* **322**, 1–11.

141. de Andres, C., Aristimuno, C., de Las Heras, V., *et al.* (2007). Interferon beta-1a therapy enhances CD4+ regulatory T-cell function: an ex vivo and in vitro longitudinal study in relapsing-remitting multiple sclerosis. *J. Neuroimmunol.* **182**, 204–211.

142. Kumar, M., Putzki, N., Limmroth, V., *et al.* (2006). CD4+CD25+FoxP3+ T lymphocytes fail to suppress myelin basic protein-induced proliferation in patients with multiple sclerosis. *J. Neuroimmunol.* **180**, 178–184.

143. Korporal, M., Haas, J., Balint, B., *et al.* (2008). Interferon beta-induced restoration of regulatory T-cell function in multiple sclerosis is prompted by an increase in newly generated naive regulatory T cells. *Arch. Neurol.* **65**, 1434–1439.

144. Hong, J., Li, N., Zhang, X., Zheng, B., and Zhang, J.Z. (2005). Induction of CD4+CD25+ regulatory T cells by copolymer-I through activation of

transcription factor Foxp3. *Proc. Natl. Acad. Sci. U. S. A.* **102**, 6449–6454.

145. Xu, L., Xu, Z., and Xu, M. (2009). Glucocorticoid treatment restores the impaired suppressive function of regulatory T cells in patients with relapsing-remitting multiple sclerosis. *Clin. Exp. Immunol.* **158**, 26–30.

146. Michel, L., Berthelot, L., Pettre, S., *et al.* (2008). Patients with relapsing-remitting multiple sclerosis have normal Treg function when cells expressing IL-7 receptor alpha-chain are excluded from the analysis. *J. Clin. Invest.* **118**, 3411–3419.

147. Fletcher, J.M., Lonergan, R., Lisa Costelloe, *et al.* (2009). CD39+Foxp3+ regulatory T cells suppress pathogenic Th17 cells and are impaired in multiple sclerosis. *J. Immunol.* **83**, 7602–7610.

148. Baecher-Allan, C.M., Costantino, C.M., Cvetanovich, G.L., *et al.* (2011). CD2 costimulation reveals defective activity by human CD4+CD25(hi) regulatory cells in patients with multiple sclerosis. *J. Immunol.* **186**, 3317–3326.

149. Fritzsching, B., Haas, J., Konig, F., *et al.* (2011). Intracerebral human regulatory T cells: analysis of CD4+ CD25+ FOXP3+ T cells in brain lesions and cerebrospinal fluid of multiple sclerosis patients. *PLoS One* **6**, e17988.

150. Schneider-Hohendorf, T., Stenner, M.P., Weidenfeller, C., *et al.* (2010). Regulatory T cells exhibit enhanced migratory characteristics, a feature impaired in patients with multiple sclerosis. *Eur. J. Immunol.* **40**, 3581–3590.

151. Malucchi, S., Sala, A., Gilli, F., *et al.* (2004). Neutralizing antibodies reduce the efficacy of betaIFN during treatment of multiple sclerosis. *Neurology* **62**, 2031–2037.

152. Ramgolam, V.S., Sha, Y., Jin, J., Zhang, X., and Markovic-Plese, S. (2009). IFN-beta inhibits human Th17 cell differentiation. *J. Immunol.* **183**, 5418–5427.

153. Sweeney, C.M., Lonergan, R., Basdeo, S.A., *et al.* (2011). IL-27 mediates the

response to IFN-beta therapy in multiple sclerosis patients by inhibiting Th17 cells. *Brain. Behav. Immun.* **25**, 1170–1181.

154. Teitelbaum, D., Meshorer, A., Hirshfeld, T., Arnon, R., and Sela, M. (1971). Suppression of experimental allergic encephalomyelitis by a synthetic polypeptide. *Eur. J. Immunol.* **1**, 242–248.

155. Comi, G., Filippi, M., and Wolinsky, J.S. (2001). European/Canadian multicenter, double-blind, randomized, placebo-controlled study of the effects of glatiramer acetate on magnetic resonance imaging: measured disease activity and burden in patients with relapsing multiple sclerosis. European/Canadian Glatiramer Acetate Study Group. *Ann. Neurol.* **49**, 290–297.

156. Kala, M., Miravalle, A., and Vollmer, T. (2011). Recent insights into the mechanism of action of glatiramer acetate. *J. Neuroimmunol.* **235**, 9–17.

157. Polman, C.H., O'Connor, P.W., Havrdova, E., et al. (2006). A randomized, placebo-controlled trial of natalizumab for relapsing multiple sclerosis. *N. Engl. J. Med.* **354**, 899–910.

158. Kappos, L., Bates, D., Hartung, H.P., et al. (2007). Natalizumab treatment for multiple sclerosis: recommendations for patient selection and monitoring. *Lancet Neurol.* **6**, 431–441.

159. Tur, C., Tintore, M., Vidal-Jordana, A., et al. (2012). Natalizumab discontinuation after PML risk stratification: outcome from a shared and informed decision. *Mult. Scler.* **Mar 1** [Epub ahead of print].

160. Kappos, L., Bates, D., Edan, G., et al. (2011). Natalizumab treatment for multiple sclerosis: updated recommendations for patient selection and monitoring. *Lancet Neurol.* **10**, 745–758.

161. Cohen, J.A. and Chun, J. (2011). Mechanisms of fingolimod's efficacy and adverse effects in multiple sclerosis. *Ann. Neurol.* **69**, 759–777.

162. Mehling, M., Lindberg, R., Raulf, F., et al. (2010). Th17 central memory T cells are reduced by FTY720 in patients with multiple sclerosis. *Neurology* **75**, 403–410.

163. Kappos, L., Radue, E.W., O'Connor, P., et al. (2010). A placebo-controlled trial of oral fingolimod in relapsing multiple sclerosis. *N. Engl. J. Med.* **362**, 387–401.

164. Cohen, J.A., Barkhof, F., Comi, G., et al. (2010). Oral fingolimod or intramuscular interferon for relapsing multiple sclerosis. *N. Engl. J. Med.* **362**, 402–415.

165. Pelletier, D. and Hafler, D.A. (2012). Fingolimod for multiple sclerosis. *N. Engl. J. Med.* **366**, 339–347.

166. Perumal, J. and Khan, O. (2012). Emerging disease-modifying therapies in multiple sclerosis. *Curr. Treat. Options Neurol.*, in press.

167. Linker, R.A., Lee, D.H., Ryan, S., et al. (2011). Fumaric acid esters exert neuroprotective effects in neuroinflammation via activation of the Nrf2 antioxidant pathway. *Brain* **134**, 678–692.

168. Ghoreschi, K., Bruck, J., Kellerer, C., et al. (2011). Fumarates improve psoriasis and multiple sclerosis by inducing type II dendritic cells. *J. Exp. Med.* **208**, 2291–2303.

169. Hill-Cawthorne, G.A., Button, T., Tuohy, O., et al. (2012). Long term lymphocyte reconstitution after alemtuzumab treatment of multiple sclerosis. *J. Neurol. Neurosurg. Psychiatry* **83**, 298–304.

170. Cossburn, M., Pace, A.A., Jones, J., et al. (2011). Autoimmune disease after alemtuzumab treatment for multiple sclerosis in a multicenter cohort. *Neurology* **77**, 573–579.

171. Kappos, L., Li, D., Calabresi, P.A., et al. (2011). Ocrelizumab in relapsing-remitting multiple sclerosis: a phase 2, randomised, placebo-controlled, multicentre trial. *Lancet* **378**, 1779–1787.

172. O'Connor, P., Wolinsky, J.S., Confavreux, C., et al. (2011). Randomized trial of oral teriflunomide for relapsing multiple sclerosis. *N. Engl. J. Med.* **365**, 1293–1303.

173. Schulze-Topphoff, U., Shetty, A., Varrin-Doyer, M., et al. (2012). Laquinimod, a

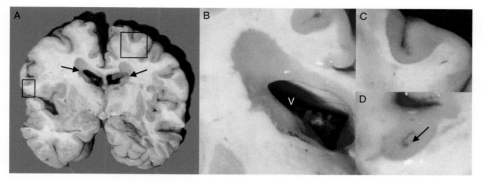

Figure 2.2. Gross pathology of MS. (A) Saggital section of the brain showing typical periventricular lesions (arrows) in MS and enlarged in (B) (v – ventricle). Boxes in (A) outline two other lesions (C) and (D). (C) is clearly a grey matter lesion impinging on a clearly demarcated lesion edge while lesion (D) centres on a blood vessel (arrow).

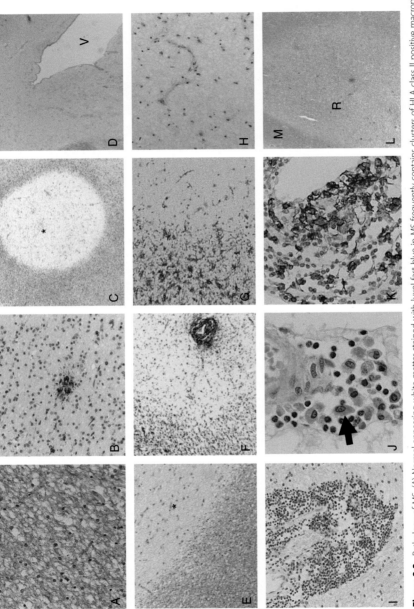

Figure 2.3. Pathology of MS. (A) Normal appearing white matter stained with luxol fast blue in MS frequently contains clusters of HLA class II positive macrophages that cluster to form a pre-active lesion (B, brown HLA class II immunohistochemistry). (C) MBP staining for demyelination, myelin (brown) shows a chronic active lesion the centre of which is devoid of myelin (*). (D) A periventricular lesion (V = ventricle) showing a large area of demyelination, LFB stain. In (E) the edge of the lesion is clearly demarcated showing normal appearing myelin (LFB stain) with the demyelinated centre (*). (F) HLA class II positive cells at the rim of a chronic active lesion and perivascular. (G) High power. (H) HLA class II positive cells at the rim of a chronic active lesion and perivascular. (I) A large perivascular cuff of T cells, B cells, and macrophages. (J) Higher power showing some of these cells are foamy macrophages that have engulfed myelin (arrow). A high proportion of these infiltrates are B cells (brown) (K). (L) A shadow plaque (pale blue area – R) surrounded by normal appearing myelin, M, representing an area of remyelination.

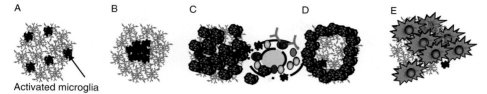

Activated microglia

Figure 2.4. Lesion progression in MS. Normal appearing white matter in MS (A) with occasional activated microglia. In the pre-active lesion, microglia migrate and form a cluster (B). An unknown trigger recruits macrophages from the blood and these cells phagocytose myelin – red globules inside the cells in an active lesion (C) and at the rim of a chronic active lesion (D). The centre of an inactive lesion is composed of hypertrophic astrocytes – the gliotic scar (E).

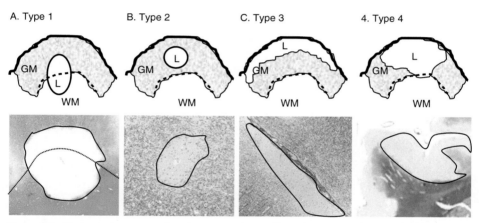

Figure 2.5. Diagrammatic representation of grey matter lesions. The representations above are diagrams showing the different grey matter lesions that depict the lesions observed in MS below. The meninges are depicted as a continuous thick black line, the edge of the lesion as a thin black line, and the border of the white and grey matter as a dotted line. GM, grey matter; WM, white matter; L demyelinated lesions.

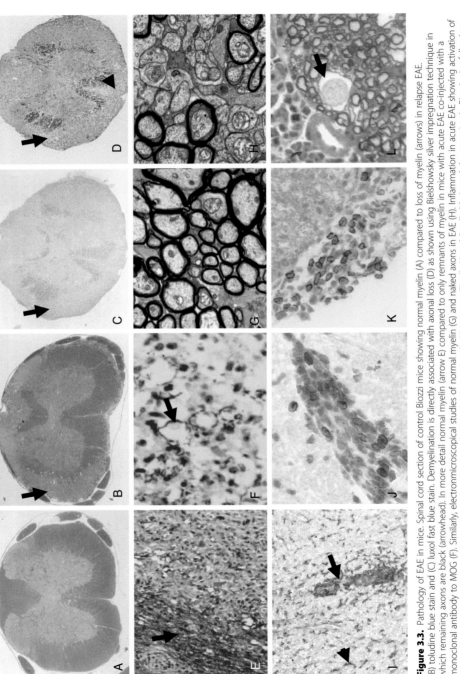

Figure 3.3. Pathology of EAE in mice. Spinal cord section of control Biozzi mice showing normal myelin (A) compared to loss of myelin (arrows) in relapse EAE. (B) toludine blue stain and (C) luxol fast blue stain. Demyelination is directly associated with axonal loss (D) as shown using Bielshowsky silver impregnation technique in which remaining axons are black (arrowhead). In more detail normal myelin (arrow E) compared to only remnants of myelin in mice with acute EAE co-injected with a monoclonal antibody to MOG (F). Similarly, electronmicroscopical studies of normal myelin (G) and naked axons in EAE (H). Inflammation in acute EAE showing activation of macrophages in the perivascular space (I, arrow) and activated microglia (I, arrowhead), CD3 positive T cells (J) and B cells (K). Axonal degeneration in Biozzi mice following immunisation with NF-L shows swollen axons (L arrow).

quinoline-3-carboxamide, induces type II myeloid cells that modulate central nervous system autoimmunity. *PLoS ONE* 7, e33797.

174. Bruck, W. and Wegner, C. (2011). Insight into the mechanism of laquinimod action. *J. Neurol. Sci.* **306**, 173–179.

175. Comi, G., Jeffery, D., Kappos, L., *et al.* (2012). Placebo-controlled trial of oral laquinimod for multiple sclerosis. *N. Engl. J. Med.* **366**, 1000–1009.

176. Esposito, F., Radaelli, M., Martinelli, V., *et al.* (2010). Comparative study of mitoxantrone efficacy profile in patients with relapsing-remitting and secondary progressive multiple sclerosis. *Mult. Scler.* **16**, 1490–1499.

177. Espejo, C. and Montalban, X. (2012). Dalfampridine in multiple sclerosis: from symptomatic treatment to immunomodulation. *Clin. Immunol.* **142**, 84–92.

Animal models based on virus infection

Gregory J. Atkins and Brian Sheahan

Animal models of MS include experimental autoimmune encephalomyelitis (EAE), and models involving infection by Theiler's virus, Semliki Forest virus and JHM coronavirus (see reference (1) for a review). The viral models utilise infection of inbred strains of laboratory mice. EAE is a non-viral model in which an MS-like disease is induced by injection of myelin components (see Chapter 3). Here the viral models will be considered, as well as models that involve the treatment of EAE by viral gene therapy.

Theiler's virus

Theiler's virus is a single-stranded RNA virus of the genus *Cardiovirus* of the family Picornaviridae. Virions have a non-enveloped icosahedral structure and contain positive-stranded RNA. After infection the genome is translated into a single polyprotein that is processed by post-translational cleavage into functional proteins. The RNA-dependent RNA polymerase, encoded by the non-structural region of the virus genome, replicates the RNA through a negative strand. Virion proteins are translated from the structural region of the viral genome, assembled with RNA into virions, and released by lysis.

Three strains of Theiler's virus have been studied: the GDVII, Daniel (DA), and BeAn strains. GDVII is neurovirulent, whereas DA and BeAn are avirulent. It is the DA and BeAn strains that have been studied as models of demyelinating disease (see references (2) and (3) for reviews). Following intracranial infection, both induce an initial grey matter disease followed by a second phase that involves virus persistence and chronic inflammatory demyelination in the white matter. In the first phase of the disease the virus infects neurons but in the second phase it infects glial cells. In susceptible mouse strains, such as SJL, the standard strain usually utilised, both phases occur, but in resistant strains, such as C57BL/6, only the first phase occurs. However, the DA and BeAn strains differ somewhat in the details and timing of the disease (4). For the BeAn strain, the early disease phase is more attenuated, in comparison to the grey matter disease induced by the DA strain. For the DA strain, the demyelinating disease is apparent at 140 to 180 days after infection whereas for the BeAn strain this occurs at 30–40 days after infection. There is approximately 100 times more virus-specific RNA in the CNS during the late phase for DA-infected mice compared to BeAn-infected mice. This correlates with more virus antigen-positive cells (microglia and oligodendrocytes) in the white matter of DA-infected as compared to BeAn-infected mice. Thus it has been concluded that the DA and BeAn strains induce distinct diseases.

The Biology of Multiple Sclerosis, ed Gregory J. Atkins, Sandra Amor, Jean M. Fletcher and Kingston H.G. Mills. Published by Cambridge University Press. © Gregory J. Atkins, Sandra Amor, Jean M. Fletcher and Kingston H.G. Mills 2012.

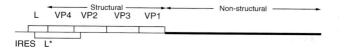

Figure 5.1. The RNA genome of Theiler's virus, shown in the 5' to 3' orientation.

Determinants of disease

The intracellular multiplication of Theiler's virus involves the translation of the entire coding region of the genome into a polyprotein, which is then processed by post-translational proteolytic cleavage into individual functional proteins (Figure 5.1).

Translation is initiated by an internal ribosome entry site (IRES): the first protein to be translated is the leader (L) protein, followed by the structural (virion) proteins, and then the non-structural (replicase) proteins. A peculiarity of the Theiler's virus genome compared to poliovirus, the prototype picornavirus, is the presence of two additional genes, L and L*, at the 5' end. The L protein is an N-terminal extension of the polyprotein, whereas the L* protein is translated out of frame compared to the polyprotein (5). Its reading frame overlaps the L/VP4/VP2 genes. Both proteins function in viral pathogenesis, but neither is required for multiplication of the virus in BHK cells in cell culture (3). In the virulent GDVII strain the AUG initiation codon of the L* protein is mutated to ACG, leading to the production of lower levels of this protein (6).

Deletions of the L protein do not affect multiplication of the DA strain of Theiler's virus in BHK cells, which do not have a functional interferon system, but they do impede the multiplication of the virus in mouse L cells, which have a functional IFN-α/β system. It has been shown that inhibition is at the transcriptional level, that the immediate early IFN genes IFN-α4 and IFN-β are inhibited, and that the mechanism is through inhibition of nucleo-cytoplasmic shuttling of the transcription factor IRF-3 (7).

Mutations in the L protein can disrupt the inhibition of interferon expression and reduce the ability of the DA strain to cause early disease and to persist (8). Thus by inhibiting interferon expression and perhaps that of other cytokines, the L protein plays an important role in pathogenesis. However, in interferon type I receptor knock-out mice the DA strain causes lethal encephalomyelitis (9). Since wild-type infected mice survive and become persistently infected, the inhibition of interferon expression cannot be absolute.

The L* protein is also involved in pathogenesis, but the mechanism is different from the L protein. Macrophages and microglial cells are important in viral pathogenesis, as they are the main reservoir during persistence (10) and also important in the immune response. In cell culture, the L* protein enhances viral replication in macrophages and microglial cells, but not in other cells. This correlates with an anti-apoptotic activity, which in turn favours persistence (11). However, the anti-apoptotic effect of the L* protein in macrophages is not absolute, and some apoptosis occurs in vivo (12). Amino acid position 93 of the L* protein has been shown to be an important determinant of both pathogenesis and demyelination (13).

Susceptibility to Theiler's virus infection (in which both phases of disease occur as opposed to just the first phase in resistant strains) maps to the H2-D locus (14, 15) of chromosome 17. The importance of the H2-D^b gene in resistance has been shown with FVB/N mice (normally susceptible) transgenic for the C57BL/6 H2-D^b gene. Such transgenic mice are resistant to persistent infection and late disease (16). Although the H2 genes exert the main effect, control of susceptibility is multigenic, and 11 other loci have been identified (3). Thus determination of the disease caused by Theiler's virus is an interplay between viral factors, in particular the L and L* genes, and multigenic control by the host.

Demyelination

Most studies of demyelination have been carried out with the SJL/J mouse strain. In the initial disease phase the virus infects mostly neurons in the grey matter, but 2 to 3 weeks after infection, there is a change in cell tropism and the virus persists in the white matter of susceptible mice, infecting macrophages, and also oligodendrocytes and astrocytes, and inducing inflammatory demyelination. The questions that can be asked, therefore, and which have not yet been fully answered, are what determines this change, and what maintains the white matter disease.

One clue to the mechanism of disease transition comes from studies of mice with myelin defects. Two important structural components of the myelin sheath surrounding axons, and formed from oligodendrocyte cytoplasmic extensions, are myelin basic protein (MBP) and proteolipid protein (PLP). Normally susceptible C3H mice with deletions or mutations in the MBP or PLP genes are resistant to persistent infection and inflammatory demyelination (17), indicating an important role for myelin in the transition process. One possible mechanism is that the virus is transported axonally from grey to white matter where it infects myelin and the oligodendrocyte cell body, and thence adjacent macrophages. This process would be blocked in mice with defective myelin (3). Immune processes are able to clear the virus from the neurons of susceptible mice, but are unable to clear it from the white matter in such mice, which leads to immune-mediated inflammatory demyelination.

Two hypotheses have been advanced to explain the mechanism of immune-mediated demyelination in Theiler's virus-induced late disease. One is epitope spreading, the other is molecular mimicry (2, 18). However, it is possible that both epitope spreading and molecular mimicry could occur during Theiler's virus-induced demyelination, since the mechanisms are not mutually exclusive. In epitope spreading, the immune reaction, initially to the virus, spreads to self components such as myelin proteins, by damage to myelin, phagocytosis, and presentation of myelin antigens.

Some myelin damage, particularly in the early stages of the disease, may occur through virus infection of oligodendrocytes. This may be due to direct killing of oligodendrocytes by the virus. Following treatment with tamoxifen, young transgenic mice that had tamoxifen-inducible expression of the DA L-coding region in oligodendrocytes showed acute progressive fatal paralysis, related to abnormalities in oligodendrocytes and demyelination, but without significant lymphocytic infiltration. Later treatment led to transient weakness with demyelination and persistent expression of the recombined transgene. These findings demonstrate that a high level of expression of DA L can cause the death of myelin-synthesising cells and death of the mouse, while a lower level of persistent L expression can lead to cellular dysfunction with survival (19). It is possible that the early infection of oligodendrocytes by the virus leads to the presentation of myelin components to the immune system.

Demyelination correlates with the presence of a CD4+ cell-mediated response to viral epitopes (20). This may in turn lead to the production of cytokines such as interferon-γ, which activate both microglial cells and macrophages. A 'bystander' effect, in which factors toxic to myelin such as tumour necrosis factor and free radicals are secreted,

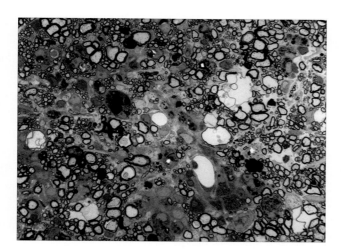

Figure 5.2. SJL mouse, 95 days after infection with the BeAn strain of Theiler's virus. Naked axons, myelin debris, vacuolated myelin sheaths, and macrophages. Toluidine Blue. Original magnification ×600.

may operate, and activated macrophages may also actively digest damaged myelin. This may lead to the presentation of myelin components to CD4+ cells, and the induction of immunity to these self antigens by epitope spreading. In SJL/J mice, the autoimmune response begins several months post inoculation, beginning with PLP epitopes, and then spreads to MBP epitopes (18).

In molecular mimicry, immune-mediated demyelination occurs by cross-reaction between self antigens and viral or other antigens, thus stimulating anti-myelin autoimmunity (1, 18). An example of molecular mimicry is that CD8+ cytotoxic T-lymphocytes specific for Theiler's virus capsid protein could recognise self protein on oligodendrocytes by molecular mimicry, leading to demyelination (21).

Semliki Forest virus

Semliki Forest virus (SFV) is a single-stranded, RNA virus of the genus *Alphavirus* of the family Togaviridae. Virions have an enveloped structure surrounding an icosahedral nucleocapsid that contains the positive-stranded RNA.

The coding region of the genome consists of a non-structural region, which encodes the replicase, and structural region, which encodes the virion proteins. During infection, the structural region is amplified by synthesis of a 26S subgenomic RNA species. The viral proteins are formed by two post-translational cleavage pathways, one of which forms the structural proteins, and the other the non-structural proteins (Figure 5.3).

SFV was first isolated in Africa and is mosquito-transmitted. It naturally infects small mammals. Virulent strains such as the L10 strain kill laboratory mice when administered peripherally, but avirulent strains such as A7 and its derivative A7[74] induce immunity but do not kill the mice. An initial observation was that virulent strains cause neuronal infection and necrosis, whereas this is less marked for avirulent strains (Figure 5.4). All strains cross the blood–brain barrier, and virulent strains cause lethal encephalomyelitis 5–7 days after infection. However, avirulent strains induce non-lethal demyelinating disease that generally lasts up to 30 days after infection (references (22–24) are reviews).

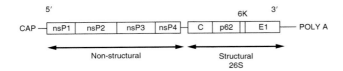

Figure 5.3. The Semliki Forest virus genome.

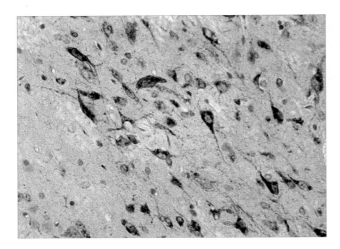

Figure 5.4. BALB/c mouse, 5 days after infection with a virulent strain of SFV. Viral antigen localised in neurons and neuronal cell processes. Anti-SFV immunohistochemistry. Original magnification ×400.

Virulence determinants

Initial studies of the determination of virulence by SFV involved the generation of mutants of the virulent L10 strain. Several mutants were isolated, and one, designated M9, had lower total RNA synthesis in cell culture than the wild-type strain. When administered peripherally, it entered the CNS and induced demyelination rather than lethal encephalitis, and infected mice survived and were immune to challenge (24). Further studies on the pathogenicity of SFV were based on comparison of the SFV4 virus, which is virulent and derived from the pSP6-SFV4 infectious clone, with the A7 or A7[74] strains. One study indicated that neurovirulence was controlled by the nsP3 gene (25), although within this gene determination was due to the accumulation of mutations (26). Other studies indicated that, although the nsP3 gene was important in the determination of virulence, an accumulation of mutations throughout the genome (27), including the 5′ untranslated region (28), was necessary for full virulence, but that deletions in the nsP3 gene attenuated virulence (29). The nsP3 gene is therefore an important virulence determinant, but it is not the only virulence determinant.

Demyelination

Following peripheral infection by avirulent SFV, a viremia is induced which lasts 3–4 days before clearance by antibody responses. The virus then crosses the blood–brain barrier and further multiplication occurs in the CNS only. The peak of virus multiplication in the CNS

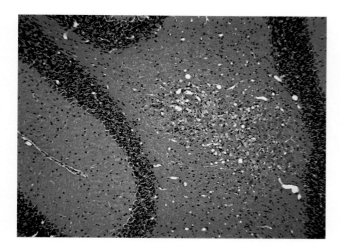

Figure 5.5. Area of demyelination in the white matter of the cerebellum of a BALB/c mouse, 14 days after intraperitoneal infection with an avirulent strain of SFV. Haematoxylin and Eosin. Original magnification ×100.

is at 5–7 days after infection, after which virus is cleared from the CNS for avirulent strains. For virulent strains, however, the virus continues to multiply and death occurs due to a lethal threshold of damage to neurons (24). Virulent strains such as L10 probably do have the capacity to induce demyelination, as shown by the effect of attenuating mutations, but this is obscured by death. For avirulent strains, the peak of inflammatory demyelination is reached at about 14 days after infection (Figures 5.5, 5.6A), when no infectious virus can be detected in the CNS, and by 20–30 days after infection in BALB/c mice, remyelination is well underway (Figure 5.6B).

Demyelination by avirulent SFV is immune-mediated, since it is much reduced in athymic (nude) mice (30, 31). Also, depletion of CD8+, but not CD4+, T cells abrogates demyelination (32). The role of antibody is, however, more controversial. Using antibody-deficient mice, one group has reported that antibody is required for viral clearance from the CNS, but is not required for demyelination (33). However, previous data using a different strain of B cell-deficient mice showed myelin vacuolation in immunocompetent but not in B cell-deficient mice, suggesting that CNS-infiltrating B cells and anti-myelin antibodies contribute to myelin injury (34). A second study (35) showed that from days 14 to 35 after infection antibodies were produced to myelin proteins. Molecular mimicry has also been described between a viral peptide and a myelin oligodendrocyte glycoprotein peptide (36).

Oligodendrocyte infection is also involved in demyelination and may be the triggering event for the immune-mediated demyelination (23; Figure 5.6C). The M9 and A7 strains show a tropism for oligodendrocytes early in infection (5–7 days) in the animal (37, 38), and a similar tropism in neural cell culture (39, 40). It has been confirmed using virus expressing fluorescently labeled protein that multiplication occurs in neurons and oligo-dendrocytes, but not in astrocytes, in the mouse CNS (41). A scheme showing the patho-genic mechanisms operating in SFV infection is shown in Figure 5.7.

Most of the studies described so far have been carried out in BALB/c mice. In this strain demyelination is followed by remyelination and does not persist. However, in the SJL mouse strain, following infection with M9-SFV, small plaques of demyelination and occasional small aggregates of mononuclear leucocytes in the leptomeninges persisted for up to 12 months.

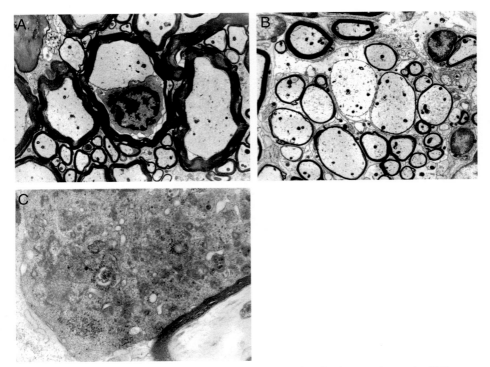

Figure 5.6. Electron micrographs of CNS tissue from BALB/c mice infected with an avirulent strain of SFV. (A) 14 days after infection. A lymphocyte interposed between an axon and a myelin sheath. Original magnification ×4500. (B) 21 days after infection. Naked axons and partially remyelinated axons with thinner than normal myelin sheaths. Original magnification ×4500. (C) 5 days after infection. Virus particles in the cytoplasm of an oligodendrocyte (note the membrane connection with a myelin sheath). Original magnification ×20 000.

This was not associated with detectable persistence of infectious virus, viral antigen, or viral RNA in the CNS (42). Also, M9-SFV infection induces long-term prolonged expression of proinflammatory cytokines (interferon-γ and tumour necrosis factor α) in the CNS of the majority of SJL (but not BALB/c) mice, which is not associated with persistence of the virus genome (43). Thus in SJL mice in this system, infection triggers a long-term inflammatory response in the CNS that is not associated with virus persistence.

Little is known regarding the mechanism of remyelination following SFV infection. However, in one study it was shown that SFV infection of $\gamma\delta$ T cell knock-out mice resulted in slower remyelination than infection of wild-type mice. Administration of a peptide epitope of the SFV envelope protein, E2 Th peptide$_2$, resulted in enhanced antibody to this peptide and also more rapid remyelination in $\gamma\delta$ T cell knock-out mice (44).

JHM coronavirus

JHM coronavirus (otherwise named mouse hepatitis virus, or MHV) is an enveloped, positive single-stranded RNA virus of the family Coronaviridae. Intracellular multiplication utilises several internal promoters on the negative strand to produce a nested

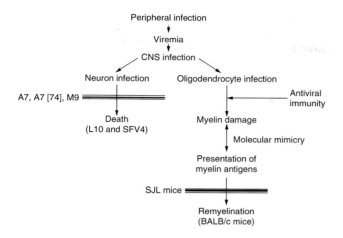

Figure 5.7. Diagrammatic representation of SFV pathogenesis. The thick lines represent partial inhibition. Following peripheral (intramuscular, intraperitoneal, or subcutaneous) infection, the virus produces a transient viremia, largely through multiplication in muscle. It then crosses the blood–brain barrier and multiplies in the CNS. All strains of SFV show a tropism for neurons and oligodendrocytes. Infection of neurons with the virulent L10 and SFV4 strains results in a lethal threshold of damage to neurons. Multiplication of the avirulent A7, A7[74], and M9 strains is partially restricted in neurons and immune intervention occurs to clear the virus before lethal damage can occur. The result of oligodendrocyte infection is myelin damage leading to the presentation of myelin antigens to the immune system and inflammatory demyelination, which could also occur by molecular mimicry. Remyelination occurs in BALB/c mice, but small lesions of demyelination and proinflammatory cytokine secretion occur in SJL mice for up to a year.

set of mRNA species, each coding for a separate protein. The negative strand is replicated by an RNA polymerase to form the positive strands that are incorporated into the virions.

In its pathogenicity in mice, JHM coronavirus shows similarities to Theiler's virus and SFV (see (45) for a review). It is neurotropic, and virulent strains such as MHV.SD cause lethal encephalitis, whereas avirulent strains such as MHV-J2.2-v1 show demyelinating disease. MHV-J2.2-v1 differs from MHV.SD by a single amino acid in the S envelope glycoprotein which recognises the viral receptor (45).

Demyelination

Demyelination occurs in MHV-J.2.2-v1 intracerebrally infected C57BL/6 mice following acute encephalitis and during the process of virus clearance. Plaques of demyelination are characterised by dense macrophage/microglial infiltration, but depletion of blood-borne macrophages does not reduce demyelination (46). Induction of demyelination is immune-mediated, since mice lacking the recombinase activating gene 1 (RAG1) or severe combined immunodeficient (SCID) mice die from encephalitis but do not show demyelination (45, 47). MHV-J.2.2-v1 infected RAG1$^{-/-}$ mice reconstituted with CD4+ and CD8+ splenocytes from MHV-immunised mice show demyelination, as do mice reconstituted with either cell type alone; however, the details of the demyelinating disease differ between cell types (48). In nude mice, demyelination does occur for MHV-J.2.2-v1 infected mice. This is because nude mice are deficient in $\alpha\beta$ T cells but not $\gamma\delta$ T cells; depletion of the latter reduces demyelination (49).

In addition to cell-mediated immunity, anti-MHV antibody also induces demyelinating disease. MHV-J.2.2-v1 infected RAG1$^{-/-}$ mice treated with anti-MHV antibody develop demyelinating disease and infiltration of white matter with macrophages/microglia (50).

Relevance to MS

The three models of virus-induced demyelination described here have similarities to each other and to MS. For all three models, both virulent and avirulent forms of the virus are available, but demyelinating disease is induced in all cases by the avirulent form. Demyelination occurs in plaques in the CNS, similar to MS, and is at least partially T cell-mediated. Macrophage/microglial infiltration is apparent, as is the case with MS.

The question therefore arises as to whether these models represent a plausible mechanism for the viral etiology of MS. The chronic demyelination associated with Theiler's virus infection is associated with virus persistence in the CNS. This is not the case with SFV and MHV-JHM, where demyelinating disease occurs during or after infectious virus clearance. Therefore this indicates two possible scenarios, either one of which is possible for MS: one is demyelinating disease associated with a persistent virus infection, the other is demyelination associated with a 'hit and run' mechanism.

Viruses as potential gene therapy agents in the treatment of MS

Modification of the possible pathogenicity of viruses and their use to treat disease rather than cause it is the basis of viral gene therapy (51). For MS this has so far been attempted in pre-clinical experiments using an animal model of MS in mice, experimental autoimmune encephalomyelitis (EAE, see Chapter 4).

Both plasmid DNA and stem cells have been used in the therapy of EAE (52). Viral gene therapy has concentrated on vectors based on herpesviruses, adenoviruses, retroviruses, vaccinia virus, and alphaviruses.

Herpesvirus vectors

Herpesviruses are large, DNA-containing viruses and vectors are based on herpes simplex virus type 1 (HSV-1), which is neurotropic (see Chapter 6). Both replication competent and non-replicative vectors have been used in the therapy of EAE. One group used a replication competent vector which had the neurovirulence $\gamma_1 34.5$ gene deleted and replaced with either IL-4 or IL-10 cytokine genes (53). It was found that intracranial injection with the IL-4-expressing vector precluded EAE, whereas no such effect was found for the IL-10-expressing vector. A later study showed that treatment with a similar vector expressing the Th2 cytokine IL-5 ameliorated EAE and decreased the numbers of infiltrating lymphocytes in the brain. This involved down-regulation of TLR 2, 3, and 9 mRNA expression and up-regulation of type I interferons in brains during onset of disease. The elevated expression of type I interferons was also seen during recovery (54).

Several studies have been carried out using a non-replicative herpesvirus vector for the treatment of EAE in mice. This vector contains a deletion of the immediate early ICP4 gene. Experiments involving a construct containing the LacZ gene inserted into the thymidine kinase locus showed that, after intracisternal injection, the virus was able to diffuse throughout the CSF and infect ependymal cells. This property has been used in studies using such a vector to express cytokine genes in the CNS (55). For example, a vector expressing the anti-inflammatory cytokine IL-4 was found to inhibit EAE (56–58). A surprising finding was that the intrathecal delivery of interferon-gamma, a proinflammatory cytokine, protected against MOG$^{33-55}$–induced EAE by increasing apoptosis of CNS-infiltrating lymphocytes (59). Intrathecal injection of a vector expressing the fibroblast growth factor-2 gene was able to inhibit chronic relapsing EAE. This was associated with an increase in the numbers of oligodendrocytes and oligodendrocyte precursors in areas of demyelination (60), indicating that remyelination may be stimulated by this treatment. Proinflammatory cytokines, such as IL-1beta, play a pathogenic role in MS and EAE. Use of a vector expressing the interleukin-1 receptor antagonist gene, a physiological antagonist of IL-1, delayed the onset of EAE (61).

These studies on murine EAE have been complemented by a study of the use of a non-replicating herpesvirus vector expressing IL-4 to treat EAE in rhesus monkeys. Intrathecal delivery of this vector was found to protect three of five monkeys from hyperacute autoimmune encephalomyelitis (62).

Adenovirus vectors

Adenoviruses are medium-sized icosahedral viruses with a linear DNA genome. The icosahedron which makes up the virion is unenveloped but has a characteristic structure consisting of fibres terminating in knobs radiating from each of the vertices. Adenovirus vectors with various parts of the genome deleted have been used extensively for gene therapy, but since they are not neurotropic, there have been relatively few studies on the CNS.

The efficacy of intrathecal adenoviral vector-mediated gene therapy in EAE in mice and the mechanism induced by IL-4 gene therapy have been demonstrated by intracisternal administration of an IL-4-producing vector (63). Mice injected with a vector expressing IL-4 showed significant clinical and neurophysiological recovery from chronic relapsing EAE. The therapeutic mechanism is probably due to increased IL-4 in the inflamed CNS areas and the ability of chemokines (CCL1, CCL17, and CCL22) to recruit CD4+ regulatory T cells.

In a further study, an adenovirus vector was used to transduce human mesenchymal stem cells (MSC) with human ciliary neurotrophic factor (CNTF; 64). CNTF had been previously found to promote myelogenesis and reduce inflammation in CNTF-deficient EAE mice. The transfected cells, which over-expressed CNTF, were injected intravenously into EAE mice 10 days after induction. Mice receiving MSC-CNTF cells showed neuronal functional recovery: the cumulative clinical scores were decreased, and the disease onset was delayed. In addition, demyelination was significantly reduced in MSC-CNTF mice. These data indicated that MSC-CNTF improved functional recovery in EAE mice, possibly by exerting their immunoregulatory activity, inhibiting inflammation, reducing demyelination, and stimulating oligodendrogenesis.

Retrovirus vectors

Retroviruses are small, RNA-containing viruses that multiply through a DNA intermediate that is integrated into the genome of the host (see Chapter 6). This property may be utilised in retrovirus vectors to transfer cloned genes to the genome of the host cell. This approach has been used to treat EAE. Cultured cells from an animal are transduced with the vector carrying the cloned gene and are then returned by transfusion (ex vivo treatment).

This approach has been used to demonstrate that T cells, transduced with a retroviral gene construct expressing IL-4, delay the onset and reduce the severity of EAE when adoptively transferred to myelin basic protein-immunised mice (65). Effector molecules such as TGF-β and nerve growth factor have also been delivered by this method and shown to be effective in ameliorating EAE (66, 67).

Brain-derived neurotrophic factor (BDNF), a pleiotrophic cytokine of the neurotrophin family, has been shown to reduce the severity of EAE (68). EAE mice receiving bone marrow stem cells (BMSCs) transduced with retrovirus containing the BDNF gene (BDNF-engineered BMSCs) were found to have delayed clinical onset and reduced clinical severity. Mice administered with BDNF-engineered BMSCs also had reduced demyelination and increased remyelination compared to mice receiving BMSC transduced with an empty vector lacking the BDNF gene (69).

A comparison has been made of the ability of retrovirus, adenovirus, and protein delivery of the anti-inflammatory cytokine IL-10 into the CNS. Fibroblasts transduced with retroviral vectors expressing IL-10 inhibited EAE, whereas an adenovirus vector expressing IL-10 and IL-10 protein at a range of doses were ineffective. It was concluded that the action of IL-10 may differ depending on the local cytokine microenvironment produced by the gene-secreting cell types (70).

Vaccinia virus vectors

Vaccinia virus is a large, enveloped DNA virus of the Poxvirus family. It is derived from the vaccine strain for human smallpox. Attenuated strains of vaccinia virus have been used in gene therapy, notably for prototype vaccine construction and inducing immune responses.

Exogenous cytokines, delivered using a recombinant vaccinia virus system, showed that IL-6, IL-1beta, IL-2, IL-10, and TNF constructs inhibited EAE whereas an IFN-gamma construct had no effect on disease; an IL-4 virus either had no effect or enhanced disease (71). Mice vaccinated with recombinant vaccinia virus encoding an encephalitogenic region of MBP were protected from EAE (72). A similar study has been carried out with marmosets induced for EAE using human white matter (73).

Alphavirus vectors

Alphaviruses are small, enveloped RNA viruses (see Chapter 2). They are naturally neurotropic. In some studies of EAE, a vector is used consisting of an avirulent strain of SFV with a multiple cloning site inserted close to the 3' end of the genome. This is therefore a replication competent vector. In other studies a virus-like particle (VLP) system is used (Figure 5.8). This consists of virus particles which are able to undergo only one round of multiplication in a host cell, but which express a cloned gene at high level in the process. Such particles cannot undergo further rounds of multiplication since they have a deletion in the viral structural genes and are therefore defective. The method of production of such recombinant VLPs is shown in Figure 5.8.

One of the problems of treating EAE with SFV vectors is that EAE is exacerbated by SFV infection at or after induction (74, 75). However, several studies have been carried out to treat EAE induced in mice with immunomodulatory genes cloned into SFV vectors. One

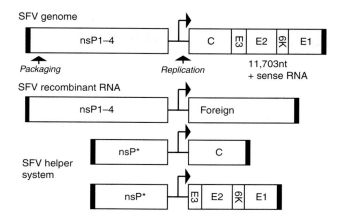

SFV genome

nsP1–4

Packaging

Replication

C | E3 | E2 | 6K | E1

11,703nt
+ sense RNA

SFV recombinant RNA

nsP1–4

Foreign

SFV helper
system

nsP*

C

nsP*

E3 | E2 | 6K | E1

Figure 5.8. The SFV recombinant particle vector system. The organisation of the wild-type SFV genome is shown at the top, above the vector and helper clones. During the multiplication of SFV, a subgenomic 26S RNA species is formed which codes for the structural proteins of the virus only, and is a gene amplification mechanism. In the SFV vector system a foreign gene is inserted in this region, in place of the viral structural proteins. RNA transcribed from this vector in vitro can be transfected by electroporation into cultured cells, and viral RNA replication and expression occur as in a productive infection. To produce recombinant particles, the packaging system is used. A helper clone has been constructed by deletion of the packaging signal, which is the RNA sequence recognised by the capsid protein for encapsidation. The viral structural proteins, which are deleted in the vector, are supplied by RNA transcribed from this helper clone, but this helper RNA is not itself packaged into capsids. Dual transfection by electroporation of helper and vector RNA results in the packaging of vector RNA into particles and their subsequent release from the cell (80).

such study utilised SFV recombinant VLPs expressing the IL-10 gene, an anti-inflammatory cytokine, administered by the intranasal route. It was shown that recombinant particles expressing the enhanced fluorescent protein (EGFP) gene or empty vector exacerbated EAE. However, those expressing IL-10 inhibited EAE. For EGFP, only the protein expressed by the gene was found in the olfactory bulb, whereas vector RNA was only found in the olfactory mucosa. It was concluded that such particles administered by the intranasal route have potential as a non-invasive vector for protein delivery to the CNS (76). In a second study, the effect of intranasal administration with SFV recombinant VLPs expressing the interferon-β (IFN-β) gene was determined. IFN-β is a cytokine used in the treatment of MS, with partially successful results. Treatment with empty vector exacerbated EAE, as did continuous treatment with IFN-β-expressing VLPs. However, IFN-β expressing recombinant VLPs, administered after induction but before the effector stage of the disease, led to an improvement in clinical and pathology score (77).

A replication competent SFV vector, based on an avirulent strain of SFV, has also been used to treat EAE. The vector was administered intraperitoneally and was neurotropic, crossing the blood–brain barrier and transferring and expressing cloned genes in the CNS. The vector was used to express tissue inhibitor of metalloproteinase (TIMP) 1–3 genes. Expression of the TIMP-2 gene significantly inhibited development of EAE. It was concluded that matrix metalloproteinases are involved in the pathogenesis of EAE (78). A similar vector has been used to treat EAE by expression of the anti-inflammatory cytokine transforming growth factor β (79).

Conclusions

Gene therapy of MS with virus vectors is still at a pre-clinical, experimental stage. No clinical trials with viral vectors have yet been carried out on MS, and so its potential cannot yet be assessed except from the available animal data.

Acknowledgements

Studies on virus-induced demyelination and virulence have been supported in our laboratories by the Multiple Sclerosis Society of Ireland, the Wellcome Trust, and the Health Research Board.

References

1. Kipp, M., van der Baukje, S., Vogel, D.Y.S., et al. (2012). Experimental in vivo and in vitro models of multiple sclerosis: EAE and beyond. *Multiple Sclerosis and Related Disorders*, **1**, 15–28.

2. Oleszak, E.L., Chang, J.R., Friedman, H., Katsetos, C.D., and Platsoucas, C.D. (2004). Theiler's virus infection: a model for multiple sclerosis. *Clin. Microbiol. Rev.* **17**, 174–207.

3. Brahic, M., Bureau, J-F., and Michiels, T. (2005). The genetics of the persistent infection and demyelinating disease caused by Theiler's virus. *Ann. Rev. Microbiol.* **59**, 279–298.

4. Zoecklein, L.J., Pavelko, K.D., Gamez, J., et al. (2003). Direct comparison of demyelinating disease induced by the Daniel's strain and BeAn strain of Theiler's murine encephalomyelitis virus. *Brain Pathol.* **13**, 291–308.

5. Kong, W.P. and Roos, R.P. (1991). Alternative translation initiation site in the DA strain of Theiler's murine encephalomyelitis virus. *J. Virol.* **65**, 3395–3399.

6. Michiels, T., Jarousse, N., and Brahic, M. (1995). Analysis of the leader and capsid coding regions of persistent and neurovirulent strains of Theiler's virus. *Virol.* **214**, 550–558.

7. Delhaye, S., van Pesch, V., and Michiels, T. (2004). The leader protein of Theiler's virus interferes with nucleocytoplasmic trafficking of cellular proteins. *J. Virol.* **78**, 4357–4362.

8. van Pesch, V., van Eyll, O., and Michiels, T. (2001). The leader protein of Theiler's virus inhibits immediate-early alpha/beta interferon production. *J. Virol.* **75**, 7811–7817.

9. Fiette, L., Aubert, C., Müller, U., et al. (1995). Theiler's virus infection of 129Sv mice that lack the interferon alpha/beta or interferon gamma receptors. *J. Exp. Med.* **181**, 2069–2076.

10. Lipton, H.L., Twaddle, G., and Jelachich, M.L. (1995). The predominant virus antigen burden is present in macrophages in Theiler's murine encephalomyelitis virus-induced demyelinating disease. *J. Virol.* **69**, 2525–2533.

11. Ghadge, G.D., Ma, L., Sato, S., Kim, J., and Roos, R.P. (1998). A protein critical for a Theiler's virus-induced immune system-mediated demyelinating disease has a cell type-specific antiapoptotic effect and a key role in persistence. *J. Virol.* **72**, 8605–8612.

12. Schlitt, B.P., Felrice, M., Jelachich, M.L., and Lipton, H.L. (2003). Apoptotic cells, including macrophages, are prominent in Theiler's virus-induced inflammatory, demyelinating lesions. *J. Virol.* **77**, 4383–4388.

13. Stavrou, S., Baida, G., Viktorova, E., Ghadge, G., Agol, V.I., and Roos, R.P. (2010). Theiler's murine encephalomyelitis virus L* amino acid position 93 is important for virus persistence and virus-induced demyelination. *J. Virol.* **84**, 1348–1354.

14. Lipton, H.L. and Melvold, R.W. (1984). Genetic analysis of susceptibility to Theiler's virus-induced demyelinating disease in mice. *J. Immunol.* **132**, 1821–1825.

15. Rodriguez, M., Leibowitz, J., and David, C.S. (1986). Susceptibility to Theiler's virus-induced demyelination. Mapping of

the gene within the H2 region. *J. Exp. Med.* **163**, 620–631.

16. Azoulay, A., Brahic, M. and Bureau J.-F. (1994). FBV mice transgenic for the H-2Db gene become resistant to persistent infection by Theiler's virus. *J. Virol.* **68**, 4049–4052.

17. Bihl, F., Pina-Rossi, C., Guénet, J-L., Brahic, M., and Bueau, J-F. (1997). The shiverer mutation affects the persistence of Theiler's virus in the central nervous system. *J. Virol.* **71**, 5025–5030.

18. Croxford, J.L., Olson, J.K., and Miller, S.D. (2002). Epitope spreading and molecular mimicry as triggers of autoimmunity in the Theiler's virus-induced demyelinating disease model of multiple sclerosis. *Autoimmun. Rev.* **1**, 251–260.

19. Ghadge, G.D., Wollman, R., Baida, G., Traka, M., and Roos, R.P. (2011). The L-coding region of the DA strain of Theiler's murine encephalomyelitis virus causes dysfunction and death of myelin-synthesizing cells. *J. Virol.* **85**, 9377–9384.

20. Gerety, S.J., Rundell, M.K., Dal Canto, M.C., and Miller, S.D. (1994). Class II-restricted T cell responses in Theiler's virus-induced demyelinating disease. VI. Potentiation of demyelination with and characterization of an immunopathologic CD4+ T cell line specific for an immunodominant VP2 epitope. *J. Immunol.* **152**, 191–929.

21. Tsunoda, I., Libbey, J.E., Kobayashi-Warren, M., and Fujinami, R.S. (2006). IFN-gamma production and astrocyte recognition by autoreactive T cells induced by Theiler's virus infection: role of viral strains and capsid proteins. *J. Neuroimmunol.* **172**, 85–93.

22. Fazakerley J.K. (2004). Semliki Forest virus infection of laboratory mice: a model to study the pathogenesis of viral encephalitis. *Arch. Virol. Suppl.* **18**, 179–190.

23. Atkins G.J., Sheahan, B.J., and Liljeström, P. (1999). The molecular pathogenesis of Semliki Forest virus: a model virus made useful? *J. Gen. Virol.* **80**, 2287–2297.

24. Atkins, G.J., Sheahan, B.J., and Dimmock, N.J. (1985). Semliki Forest virus infection of mice: a model for genetic and molecular analysis of viral pathogenicity. *J. Gen. Virol.* **66**, 395–408.

25. Tuittila, M.T., Santagati, M.G., Röyttä, M., Määttä, J.A., and Hinkkanen, A.E. (2000). Replicase complex genes of Semliki Forest virus confer lethal neurovirulence. *J. Virol.* **74**, 4579–4589.

26. Tuittila, M. and Hinkkanen, A.E. (2003). Amino acid mutations in the replicase protein nsP3 of Semliki Forest virus cumulatively affect neurovirulence. *J. Gen. Virol.* **84**, 1525–1533.

27. Tarbatt, C.J., Glasgow, G.M., Mooney, D.A., Sheahan, B.J., and Atkins, G.J. (1997). Sequence analysis of the avirulent, demyelinating A7 strain of Semliki Forest virus. *J. Gen. Virol.* **78**, 1551–1557.

28. Logue, CH, Sheahan, B.J., and Atkins G.J. (2008). The 5' untranslated region as a pathogenicity determinant of Semliki Forest virus in mice. *Virus Genes* **36**, 313–321.

29. Galbraith, S.E., Sheahan, B.J., and Atkins, G.J. (2006). Deletions in the hypervariable domain of the nsP3 gene attenuate Semliki Forest virus virulence. *J. Gen. Virol.* **87**, 937–947.

30. Gates, M.C., Sheahan, B.J., and Atkins, G.J. (1984). The pathogenicity of the M9 mutant of Semliki Forest virus in immune-compromised mice. *J. Gen. Virol.* **65**, 73–80.

31. Fazakerley, J.K. and Webb, H.E. (1987). Semliki Forest virus-induced, immune-mediated demyelination: adoptive transfer studies and viral persistence in nude mice. *J. Gen. Virol.* **68**, 377–385.

32. Subak-Sharpe, I., Dyson, H., and Fazakerley, J. (1993). In vivo depletion of CD8+ T cells prevents lesions of demyelination in Semliki Forest virus infection. *J. Virol.* **67**, 7629–7633.

33. Fragkoudis, R., Ballany, C.M., Boyd, A., and Fazakerley, J.K. (2008). In Semliki Forest virus encephalitis, antibody rapidly clears infectious virus and is required to eliminate viral material from the brain, but is not required to generate lesions of

demyelination. *J. Gen. Virol.* **89**, 2565–2568.

34. Smith-Norowitz, T.A., Sobel, R.A., and Mokhtarian, F. (2000). B cells and antibodies in the pathogenesis of myelin injury in Semliki Forest Virus encephalomyelitis. *Cell Immunol.* **200**, 27–35.

35. Mokhtarian, F., Huan C.M., Roman, C., and Raine, C.S. (2003). Semliki Forest virus-induced demyelination and remyelination – involvement of B cells and anti-myelin antibodies. *J. Neuroimmunol.* **137**, 19–31.

36. Mokhtarian, F., Zhang Z., Shi, Y., Gonzales, E., and Sobel, R.A. (1999). Molecular mimicry between a viral peptide and a myelin oligodendrocyte glycoprotein peptide induces autoimmune demyelinating disease in mice. *J. Neuroimmunol.* **95**, 43–54.

37. Sheahan, B.J., Gates, M.C., Caffrey, J.F., and Atkins, G.J. (1983). Oligodendrocyte infection and demyelination produced in mice by the M9 mutant of Semliki Forest virus. *Acta Neuropathol.* **60**, 257–265.

38. Gates, M.C., Sheahan, B.J., and Atkins, G.J. (1984). The pathogenicity of the M9 mutant of Semliki Forest virus in immune compromised mice. *J. Gen. Virol.* **65**, 73–80.

39. Gates, M.C., Sheahan, B.J., O'Sullivan, M.A., and Atkins, G.J. (1985). Pathogenicity of the A7, M9 and L10 strains of Semliki Forest virus for weanling mice and primary mouse brain cell cultures. *J. Gen. Virol.* **66**, 2365–2373.

40. Atkins, G.J., Sheahan, B.J., and Mooney, D.A. (1990). Pathogenicity of Semliki Forest virus for the rat central nervous system and primary rat neural cell cultures: possible implications for the pathogenesis of multiple sclerosis. *Neuropath. Appl. Neurobiol.* **16**, 57–68.

41. Fragkoudis, R., Tamberg, N., Siu, R., *et al.* (2009). Neurons and oligodendrocytes in the mouse brain differ in their ability to replicate Semliki Forest virus. *J. Neurovirol.* **15**, 57–70.

42. Smyth, J.M., Sheahan, B.J., and Atkins, G.J. (1990). Multiplication of virulent and demyelinating Semliki Forest virus in the mouse central nervous system: consequences in BALB/c and SJL mice. *J. Gen. Virol.* **71**, 2575–2583.

43. Donnelly, S.M., Sheahan, B.J., and Atkins, G.J. (1997). Long-term effects of Semliki Forest virus infection in the mouse central nervous system. *Neuropathol. Appl. Neurobiol.* **23**, 235–241.

44. Safavi, F., Feliberti, J.P., Raine, C.S., and Mokhtarian, F. (2011). Role of γδ T cells in antibody production and recovery from SFV demyelinating disease. *J. Neuroimmunol.* **235**, 18–26.

45. Templeton, S.P. and Perlman, S. (2007). Pathogenesis of acute and chronic central nervous system infection with variants of mouse hepatitis virus, strain JHM. *Immunol. Res.* **39**, 160–172.

46. Xue, S., Sun, N., van Rooijen, N., and Perlman, S. (1999). Depletion of blood-borne macrophages does not reduce demyelination in mice infected with a neurotropic coronavirus. *J. Virol.* **73**, 6327–6334.

47. Houtman, J.J. and Fleming, J.O. (1996). Pathogenesis of mouse hepatitis virus-induced demyelination. *J. Neurovirol.* **2**, 361–376.

48. Wu, G.F., Dandekar, A.A., Pewe, L., and Perlman, S. (2000). CD4 and CD8 T cells redundant but not identical roles in virus-induced demyelination. *J. Immunol.* **165**, 2278–2286.

49. Dandekar, A.A. and Perlman, S. (2002). Virus-induced demyelination in nude mice is mediated by gamma delta T cells. *Am. J. Pathol.* **1611**, 1255–1263.

50. Kim, T.S. and Perlman, S. (2005). Virus-specific antibody, in the absence of T cells, mediates demyelination in mice infected with a neurotropic coronavirus. *Am. J. Pathol.* **166**, 801–809.

51. Kay, M.A., Glorioso, J.C., and Naldini, L. (2001). Viral vectors for gene therapy: the art of turning infectious agents into vehicles of therapeutics. *Nat. Med.* **7**, 33–40.

52. Leung, P.S.C., Shu, S., Kenny, T.P., Wu, P., and Tao M. (2010). Development and validation of gene therapies in autoimmune diseases: epidemiology to animal models. *Autoimmun. Rev.* **9**, 400–405.

53. Broberg E, Setala N., Roytta, M., et al. (2001). Expression of interleukin-4 but not of interleukin-10 from a replicative herpes simplex virus type 1 viral vector precludes experimental allergic encephalomyelitis. *Gene Ther.* **8**, 769–777.

54. Nygårdas, M., Aspelin, C., Paavilainen, H., Röyttä, M., Waris, M., and Hukkanen, V. (2011). Treatment of experimental autoimmune encephalomyelitis in SJL/J mice with a replicative HSV-1 vector expressing interleukin-5. *Gene Ther.* **18**, 646–655.

55. Martino, G., Poliani, P.L., Marconi, P.C., Comi, G., and Furlan, R. (2000). Cytokine gene therapy of autoimmune demyelination revisited using herpes simplex virus type-1-derived vectors. *Gene Ther.* **7**, 1087–1093.

56. Martino, G., Furlan, R., Galbiati, F., et al. (1998). A gene therapy approach to treat demyelinating diseases using non-replicative herpetic vectors engineered to produce cytokines. *Mult. Scler.* **4**, 222–227.

57. Furlan, R., Poliani, P.L., Galbiati, F., et al. (1998). Central nervous system delivery of interleukin-4 by a non-replicative herpes simplex type 1 viral vector ameliorates autoimmune demyelination. *Hum. Gene Ther.* **9**, 2605–2617.

58. Furlan, R., Poliani, P.L., Marconi, P.C., et al. (2001). Central nervous system gene therapy with interleukin-4 inhibits progression of ongoing relapsing-remitting autoimmune encephalomyelitis in Biozzi AB/H mice. *Gene Ther.* **8**, 13–19.

59. Furlan R., Brambilla E., Ruffini F., et al. (2001). Intrathecal delivery of IFN-gamma protects C57BL/6 mice from chronic-progressive experimental autoimmune encephalomyelitis by increasing apoptosis of central nervous system-infiltrating lymphocytes. *J. Immunol.* **167**, 1821–1829.

60. Ruffini, F., Furlan, R., Poliani, P.L., et al. (2001). Fibroblast growth factor-II gene therapy reverts the clinical course and the pathological signs of chronic experimental autoimmune encephalomyelitis in C57BL/6 mice. *Gene Ther.* **8**, 1207–1213.

61. Furlan, R., Bergami, A., Brambilla, E., et al. (2007). HSV-1-mediated IL-1 receptor antagonist gene therapy ameliorates MOG (35–55)-induced experimental autoimmune encephalomyelitis in C57BL/6 mice. *Gene Ther.* **14**, 93–98.

62. Poliani, P.L., Brok, H., Furlan, R., et al. (2001). Delivery to the central nervous system of a nonreplicative herpes simplex type 1 vector engineered with the interleukin 4 gene protects rhesus monkeys from hyperacute autoimmune encephalomyelitis. *Hum. Gene Ther.* **12**, 905–920.

63. Butti, E., Bergami, A., Recchia, A., et al. (2008). IL4 gene delivery to the CNS recruits regulatory T cells and induces clinical recovery in mouse models of multiple sclerosis. *Gene Ther.* **15**, 504–515.

64. Lu, Z., Hu, X., Zhu, C., Wang, D., Zheng, X., and Liu, Q. (2009). Overexpression of CNTF in mesenchymal stem cells reduces demyelination and induces clinical recovery in experimental autoimmune encephalomyelitis mice. *J. Neuroimmunol.* **206**, 58–69.

65. Shaw, M.K., Lorens, J.B., Dhawan, A., et al. (1997). Local delivery of interleukin 4 by retrovirus-transduced T lymphocytes ameliorates experimental autoimmune encephalomyelitis. *J. Exp. Med.* **185**, 1711–1714.

66. Chen, L.Z., Hochwald, G.M., Huang, C., et al. (1998). Gene therapy in allergic encephalomyelitis using myelin basic protein-specific T cells engineered to express latent transforming growth factor-beta1. *Proc. Natl. Acad. Sci. U.S.A.* **95**, 12516–12521.

67. Flugel, A., Matsumuro, K., Neumann, H., et al. (2001). Anti-inflammatory activity of nerve growth factor in experimental autoimmune encephalomyelitis: inhibition of monocyte transendothelial migration. *Eur. J. Immunol.* **31**, 11–22.

68. Makar, T.K., Trisler, D., Sura, K.T., Sultana, S., Patel, N., and Bever, C.T. (2008). Brain derived neurotrophic factor treatment reduces inflammation and apoptosis in experimental allergic encephalomyelitis. *J. Neurol. Sci.* **270**, 70–76.

69. Makar, T.K., Bever, C.T., Singh, I.S., *et al.* (2009). Brain-derived neurotrophic factor gene delivery in an animal model of multiple sclerosis using bone marrow stem cells as a vehicle. *J. Neuroimmunol.* **210**, 40–51.

70. Croxford, J.L., Feldmann, M., Chernajovsky, Y., and Baker, D. (2001). Different therapeutic outcomes in experimental allergic encephalomyelitis dependent upon the mode of delivery of IL-10: a comparison of the effects of protein, adenoviral or retroviral IL-10 delivery into the central nervous system. *J. Immunol.* **166**, 4124–4130.

71. Willenborg, D.O., Fordham, S.A., Cowden, W.B., and Ramshaw, I.A. (1995). Cytokines and murine autoimmune encephalomyelitis: inhibition or enhancement of disease with antibodies to select cytokines, or by delivery of exogenous cytokines using a recombinant vaccinia virus system. *Scand. J. Immunol.* **41**, 31–41.

72. Barnett, L.A., Whitton, J.L., Wang, L.Y., and Fujinami, R.S. (1996). Virus encoding an encephalitogenic peptide protects mice from experimental allergic encephalomyelitis. *J. Neuroimmunol.* **64**, 163–173.

73. Genain, C.P., Gritz, L., Joshi, N., *et al.* (1997). Inhibition of allergic encephalomyelitis in marmosets by vaccination with recombinant vaccinia virus encoding for myelin basic protein. *J. Neuroimmunol.* **79**, 119–128.

74. Wu, L.X., Mäkelä, M.J., Röyttä, M., and Salmi, A. (1988). Effect of viral infection on experimental allergic encephalomyelitis in mice. *J. Neuroimmunol.* **18**, 139–153.

75. Erälinna, J.P., Soilu-Hänninen, M., Röyttä, M., Ilonen, J., Mäkelä, A., and Salonen, R. (1994). Facilitation of experimental allergic encephalomyelitis by irradiation and virus infection: role of inflammatory cells. *J. Neuroimmunol.* **55**, 81–90.

76. Jerusalmi, A., Morris-Downes, M.M., Sheahan, B.J., and Atkins, G.J. (2003). Effect of intranasal administration of Semliki Forest virus recombinant particles expressing reporter and cytokine genes on the progression of experimental autoimmune encephalomyelitis. *Mol. Ther.* **8**, 886–894.

77. Quinn K., Galbraith, S.E., Sheahan, B.J., and Atkins, G.J. (2008). Effect of intranasal administration of Semliki Forest virus recombinant particles expressing interferon-β on the progression of experimental autoimmune encephalomyelitis. *Mol. Med. Reports* **1**, 335–342.

78. Nygårdas, P.T., Grönberg, S.A., Heikkilä, J., Joronen, K., Sorsa, T., and Hinkkanen, A.E. (2004). Treatment of experimental autoimmune encephalomyelitis with a neurotropic alphavirus vector expressing tissue inhibitor of metalloproteinase-2. *Scand. J. Immunol.* **60**, 372–381.

79. Vähä-Koskela, M.J., Kuusinen, T.I., Holmlund-Hampf, J.C., Furu, P.T., Heikkilä, J.E., and Hinkkanen, A.E. (2007). Semliki Forest virus vectors expressing transforming growth factor beta inhibit experimental autoimmune encephalomyelitis in Balb/c mice. *Biochem. Biophys. Res. Commun.* **355**, 776–781.

80. Smerdou, C. and Liljeström, P. (1999). Two-helper RNA system for production of recombinant Semliki Forest virus particles. *J. Virol.* **73**, 1092–1098.

Viruses in the etiology of MS

6

Gregory J. Atkins

Studies of the epidemiology and genetics of MS suggest an interaction between an environ-mental factor and genetic susceptibility (see Chapter 1). Several animal and human infec-tions show CNS demyelination, which may be at least partially autoimmune. For this reason, virus infection has been implicated in the etiology of MS. Several viruses have been implicated, but the evidence in all cases is equivocal. Here the evidence linking the various candidate viruses is summarised.

Measles and rubella viruses

Measles virus is a member of the genus *Morbillivirus* of the family Paramyxoviridae. It is a negative-stranded, enveloped RNA virus. Because of its association with rare demyelinating diseases in man, and the association of other morbilliviruses with demyelinating disease in animals, it has long been considered a candidate in the etiology of MS (reference (1) is a review of the pathogenesis of morbilliviruses). Measles virus is a component of the live attenuated measles-mumps-rubella (MMR) vaccine that is in universal use in developed countries and has led to a substantial decrease in the incidence of these diseases.

Rubella virus has also been implicated in the etiology of MS. It is the sole member of the genus *Rubivirus* of the family Togaviridae (reference (2) is a review of the pathogenicity of rubella virus). It is a positive-stranded, enveloped RNA virus and has a multiplication strategy and structure similar to Semliki Forest virus (see Chapter 5).

The third component of the MMR vaccine is mumps virus, which like measles virus is a negative-stranded RNA virus of the family Paramyxoviridae. It has not been implicated in MS, except in the context that, along with several other pathogens, later infections increase the risk of MS (3), a hypothesis that has been refuted (4).

Characteristics of the viruses

The genome of measles virus is shown in Figure 6.1. Like other negative-stranded RNA viruses, the virion contains an RNA polymerase (the L protein) that transcribes the negative-stranded genome on infection into positive-stranded RNA.

Before the advent of the MMR vaccine, measles was a common childhood infection. It is now rare in developed countries, although still common in the developing world. There is only one serotype, so infection confers life-long immunity. The disease is aerosol

The Biology of Multiple Sclerosis, ed Gregory J. Atkins, Sandra Amor, Jean M. Fletcher and Kingston H.G. Mills. Published by Cambridge University Press. © Gregory J. Atkins, Sandra Amor, Jean M. Fletcher and Kingston H.G. Mills 2012.

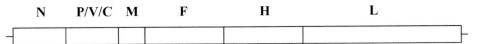

Figure 6.1. Structure of the measles virus genome. The negative-stranded RNA genome is shown in the 3′ to 5′ orientation. N is the nucleocapsid protein, P is a phospholipid protein associated with the nucleocapsid, M is the matrix protein that underlies the envelope, F and H are the fusion and haemagglutinin envelope proteins, and L is a large protein that functions as the virion polymerase. V and C are non-structural proteins generated from a reading frame overlapping the P gene.

transmitted, and is highly contagious. The virus initially multiplies in the upper respiratory tract, and then progresses to cells of the immune system, which disseminates the virus (1). Infection with measles produces immunosuppression in the host, which derives from several viral proteins, lasts up to 6 months after infection, and increases susceptibility to secondary infection (5). The symptoms of acute measles infection are preceded by characteristic spots on the mucosal surface of the mouth, called Koplik spots. This is followed by a maculopapular rash, dry cough, coryza, fever, conjunctivitis, and photophobia (1).

There are three serious complications of measles virus infection, all of which involve the CNS and are associated with demyelination. These are acute disseminated encephalomyelitis (ADEM), measles inclusion body encephalitis (MIBE), and subacute sclerosing panencephalitis (SSPE).

Rubella virus causes a normally mild infection in man, triggering a maculopapular rash in less than 50% of cases; infections are often subclinical, and it is aerosol transmitted (6, 7). Other symptoms can include lymphadenopathy, fever, conjunctivitis, sore throat, and arthralgia. Initial sites of virus replication are the mucosa of the upper respiratory tract and nasopharyngeal lymphoid tissue. From here the virus becomes viremic and spreads to lymphoid and other tissue.

A complication of rubella virus infection is congenital rubella syndrome (6). This occurs when a pregnant woman is infected during the first 3 months of pregnancy and the virus traverses the placenta. A chronic infection of the foetus follows in 90% of cases and the virus is teratogenic. The introduction of the MMR vaccine has greatly reduced the incidence of the disease. The infant is born with a chronic rubella infection, and birth defects include cloudy cornea, deafness, developmental delay, low birth weight, mental retardation, seizures, small head size, and a skin rash.

Progressive rubella panencephalitis (PRP) is a CNS complication of rubella virus infection.

Acute disseminated encephalomyelitis

ADEM is a rare complication of measles virus infection that also occurs with other pathogens (8); it has also been seen following measles vaccination. It occurs in 1/1000 infected children and has a 20% mortality. Symptoms occur after the initial rash and are neurological, consisting of seizures and multifocal neurological signs. Demyelination occurs similar to MS. MRI indicates newly developed multifocal white matter lesions. Measles virus has not been isolated from the brain and the link with the virus infection is suggested by the close temporal relationship between infection or vaccination and neurological signs.

Measles inclusion body encephalitis

MIBE occurs several months after measles infection or vaccination, in immunocompromised hosts (1, 9). It is fatal in 78% of cases, with survivors retaining a persistent neurological disease. Measles virus RNA or protein can be detected in autopsy samples, by RT-PCR or immunohistochemistry. Neuropathological examination shows focal necrosis, glial cell proliferation, and often intracellular inclusion bodies and axonal demyelination.

Subacute sclerosing panencephalitis

SSPE is a rare neurological disease, occurring in one in 10 000–25 000 children after measles infection, and about 5–10 years after the initial acute infection (1, 9). It is a chronic defective CNS infection, but it is not known where the virus resides during the years of latency. Children present with neurological symptoms that gradually degenerate to a vegetative state, followed by death. Although typical viral inclusions are found in neurons, and to a lesser extent oligodendrocytes and astrocytes, infectious virus cannot be isolated from the CNS at autopsy.

High antibody titres to the measles virus structural proteins N, F, and H are found in both the blood and cerebrospinal fluid (CSF), with intrathecally synthesised oligoclonal bands (10). In addition, there is a widespread lymphocytic infiltration, and the white matter shows focal demyelination and astrogliosis. These signs are also characteristic of MS.

Progressive rubella panencephalitis

PRP is a disease like SSPE and has a lower incidence (2). It occurs several years after acute rubella infection or congenital infection. Elevated CSF total protein and globulin and elevated rubella antibodies in CSF and serum occur. Infectious rubella virus cannot be recovered. PRP has many clinical, neuropathological, and immunological similarities to SSPE, including white matter lesions, suggesting that both diseases may have common pathogenetic factors (11).

Link with MS?

Suspicions that measles and/or rubella viruses may be linked with MS were initially based on the capability of the viruses to induce demyelination, as described above, and the presence of antibody in the blood and CSF of MS patients. For example, one group has found antibody primarily to the measles virus N protein in the CSF of MS patients (12). It has been found that the antibody response to the rubella virus envelope glycoprotein E2 is elevated in MS patients (13). Antibodies to canine distemper virus, a neurotropic canine morbillivirus closely related to measles virus, have been linked to MS (14). However, it is clear that measles and canine distemper antibodies cross-react. Most patients with MS display a polyspecific, intrathecal humoral immune response against a broad panel of viral agents including antibodies to measles, rubella, and varicella-zoster viruses as the three most abundant components; this is called the MRZ reaction (15). However, it is not known whether this is related to the etiology of MS, a result of MS, or a result of CNS autoimmunity in general.

Two searches have been carried out to detect measles and other virus RNA sequences in the tissues of MS patients, with equivocal results. In one study (16), CNS samples from eight MS cases and 56 controls were examined for sequences of measles virus, canine distemper virus, simian virus 5 (a simian paramyxovirus once associated with

MS), and rubella virus by in situ hybridisation using RNA probes. Foci of hybridisation were found in two of the MS cases using probes against the measles virus N protein, the P protein, and the F protein, and also in one control. No hybridisation was found in any other instance. In a separate study, peripheral blood leucocytes from 17 MS patients, healthy controls, and one acute measles case were examined for measles virus RNA using the reverse transcription polymerase chain reaction. Only the acute measles virus sample was positive (17). Thus it is clear that MS is not usually associated with the persistence of measles virus RNA, either in peripheral leucocytes or in the CNS. However, this does not exclude the possibility of a transient virus infection that could act as a trigger for MS.

The MMR vaccine has been implicated in the etiology of MS since it consists of a mixture of the three live attenuated viruses, and childhood infections have been implicated in MS pathogenesis. One study found no vaccination-related MS incidence changes (18). However, this does not exclude the possibility that MS could be triggered in a minority of vaccine recipients and cause a minority of cases of MS (19), since MS is a heterologous disease (20).

Herpesviruses

Herpesviruses are large, enveloped DNA viruses that infect both man and animals. They multiply in the nucleus of infected cells, acquiring their envelope from the nuclear membrane. The DNA typically codes for 100–200 genes, and transcription and translation of the genome occurs by a cascade mechanism. There are eight types or species of human herpesvirus, but only five of these have been associated with MS. These are herpes simplex virus (HSV) types 1 and 2, varicella-zoster virus (VZV), human herpesvirus type 6 (HHV-6), and Epstein–Barr virus (EBV)(21). Marek's disease virus, a herpes disease primarily of birds, has been associated with a cluster of MS cases in Key West, Florida (22).

Herpesviruses typically show latency, i.e. the virus can enter a non-infectious state for months or years, and then reappear and cause disease symptoms. During the latent period, the virus expresses only some early genes, termed latency-associated transcripts. Examples of latency include HSV type 1 and cold sores around the mouth, VZV (chickenpox) and zoster (shingles), and EBV, which is latent in B-lymphocytes. Both HSV-1 and VZV are latent in neurons in nerve ganglia (23).

Herpes simplex viruses type 1 and 2

It has been postulated that MS could be triggered by infection with HSV-2 in individuals lacking immunity to HSV-1 (24), but there is no definitive evidence to support this hypothesis.

HSV-1 DNA and RNA have been found in a proportion of acute MS patients in peripheral blood mononuclear cells but not in normal controls, using nested PCR (25). This indicates that HSV-1 re-activates during relapses and could act as a trigger. Equally, HSV-1 activation could be a result of the relapse.

Varicella-zoster virus

As indicated in Chapter 3, most MS patients display a polyspecific, intrathecal humoral immune response against measles, rubella, and VZV, the MRZ reaction (26). One study revealed a high frequency of VZV DNA in the CSF of patients with MS compared to other neurological diseases or normal controls (27). A subsequent study associated the activation of VZV with relapses of MS. Particles with the morphology of VZV were found in CSF from MS patients within the first few days of a relapse, but were not found in patients in remission or in controls. Also, VZV DNA was found by real-time PCR in CSF and in peripheral blood mononuclear cells during relapse, disappearing in most patients during remission (28). These results may suggest a possible role of this virus in the pathogenesis of MS, or may indicate that the virus is activated in MS patients as a consequence of the disease, particularly during relapse (29).

However, a more recent study found no herpesvirions or VZV DNA in MS CSF during relapses or in acute MS plaques, using the same electron microscopic techniques and primers (plus additional primers) as the previous study. Although enzyme-linked immuno-sorbent assay showed a higher titre of VZV antibody in MS CSF than in control samples, recombinant antibodies prepared from clonally expanded MS CSF plasma cells did not bind to VZV. The authors therefore concluded that VZV is not a disease-relevant antigen in MS (30). Thus there are conflicting studies concerning the presence of VZV DNA and antigen in the CSF of relapsing MS patients.

Human herpesvirus type 6

HHV-6 was first isolated from patients with lymphoproliferative disorders, but is now known to be neurotropic. Two variants have been identified, labeled HHV-6A and HHV-6B, which share 90% sequence homology. HHV-6B causes a common childhood disease termed exanthema subitum, also known as roseola, which is characterised by a high fever and rash. Attempts at association of HHV-6 with MS have involved both variants.

Many reports have now been published describing attempts to associate HHV-6 with MS. The main problem has been showing an association between what appears to be a ubiquitous virus and MS. Most studies are based on detection of antibodies in the serum or CSF, or amplification of HHV-6 DNA by PCR from sera or CSF of MS patients. Some studies have detected HHV-6 DNA in MS plaques. In their 2005 review, Fotheringham and Jacobson (31) found that five out of nine studies measuring serum HHV-6 IgM levels indicated active HHV-6 infection in MS patients, whereas one out of four detected IgM in CSF. High levels of serum HHV-6 IgG are detected in MS patients, but this is also detected in controls. HHV-6 DNA has been found in the serum, peripheral blood mononuclear cells, CSF, and brain. However, this DNA has also been detected in control tissue in several studies (31).

In their study of MS and control brains by laser microdissection, Cermelli et al. (32) found a higher frequency of human herpes 6 DNA in MS plaques, and concluded that HHV-6 may play a role in pathogenesis. However, a negative result has been found by Mameli et al. (33), who found that there were no significant differences between MS patients and controls for HHV-6 presence and replication in the brain or in peripheral blood mononuclear cells.

Molecular mimicry has been postulated to explain the possible role of HHV-6 in the pathogenesis of MS. Two studies have shown cross-reactivity between myelin basic protein (MBP) and HHV-6 viral antigen (34, 35). In particular, one study identified the 1–13 region of a viral protein, U34, as showing homology with the 93–105 region of human MBP. Thus active replication of HHV-6 in MS patients may sensitise the immune system to this region of MBP and may increase sensitivity to other MBP epitopes by epitope spreading (35).

Epstein–Barr virus

EBV is a ubiquitous pathogen that infects more than 90% of the world's population. It is B-lymphotropic and shows life-long latency in B cells, being occasionally re-activated in some individuals and spreading through the saliva. Childhood infections are usually asymptomatic, whereas infection at or after adolescence results in symptoms of infectious mononucleosis in about half of cases.

Many serological studies have been carried out to investigate the relationship between EBV immunity and MS (reviewed in (36)). Serological data, mainly against the EBV viral capsid antigen or EBV nuclear antigen (EBNA), consistently show a close to 100% EBV seropositivity rate in MS patients and elevated titres.

Infectious mononucleosis is more common in adolescence and adults than it is in children, where the infection is usually clinically silent. It shows the same geographical distribution as MS, i.e. shows a latitude prevalence with increasing distance north and south of the equator (36). Epidemiological studies involving large numbers of patients have concluded that the risk for MS is close to zero for EBV-negative individuals, intermediate among those infected in childhood, and highest among those infected later in life (37).

One study investigated expression of EBV markers in autopsy brain tissue from MS cases with different clinical courses (38). They found evidence of EBV infection in a substantial proportion of brain-infiltrating B cells and plasma cells. Ectopic B cell follicles forming in the cerebral meninges of some cases with secondary progressive MS were identified as major sites of EBV persistence. Expression of viral latent proteins was observed in MS brains, whereas viral re-activation appeared restricted to ectopic B cell follicles and acute lesions. These findings were interpreted as evidence that EBV persistence and reactivation in the CNS play an important role in MS immunopathology. However, two further studies have failed to confirm these results. To assess whether EBV infection is a characteristic feature of MS brain, a large cohort of MS specimens containing white matter lesions (nine adult and three paediatric cases) with a heterogeneous B cell infiltrate and a second cohort of MS specimens (12 cases) that included B cell infiltration within the meninges and parenchymal B cell aggregates were examined for EBV infection using multiple methodologies including in situ hybridisation, immunohistochemistry, and two independent real-time polymerase chain reaction (PCR) methodologies (39). EBV could not be detected in any of the MS specimens by any of the methods, except for two specimens where low levels of EBV RNA could be detected by RT-PCR. This indicates that EBV infection is unlikely to contribute directly to MS brain pathology in the vast majority of cases. Using similar techniques, a second negative study showed that abundant EBV infection of the CNS is unlikely to contribute to the later stages of the pathogenesis of MS (40). However, whether or not EBV acts earlier in the course of disease, perhaps as a trigger, or activating and perpetuating inflammation, cannot be excluded by either of these studies.

Intrathecal production of IgG occurs in both MS and CNS infections (41). There are several reports of an anti-EBV immune response in the CNS of MS patients (36). However, this occurs for several other pathogens also (26). Also, the frequency of, and proliferative capacity of, EBNA 1-specific T cells has been found to be elevated in MS patients (42).

Cross-reactive T cells between EBV peptides and myelin proteins, including myelin basic protein, have been detected, although at similar frequency in MS patients and controls. Nevertheless, this has led to the proposal of autoimmunity by molecular mimicry for EBV (43).

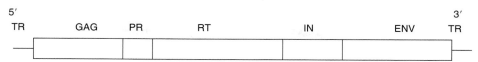

Figure 6.2. Basic structure of the retrovirus genome. TR, terminal repeat; GAG, nucleocapsid protein gene; PR, protease; RT, reverse transcriptase; IN, integrase; ENV, envelope protein.

Conclusions

Herpesviruses show life-long latent infection, and re-activation could result in periodic challenge to the immune system, and possibly trigger a chronic inflammatory immune response as seen in MS. However, an opposite argument can also be made, i.e. that the inflammatory immune response as seen in MS leads to the re-activation of latent herpesviruses. At present these two possibilities cannot be differentiated. Association between serum and/or CNS antibodies is subject to the same argument; association does not indicate causation.

For HHV-6 and EBV, molecular mimicry has been postulated to play a role in disease pathogenesis. However, there is little direct mechanistic evidence to substantiate this, although it remains an intriguing possibility.

Retroviruses

Retroviruses are enveloped RNA-containing viruses that replicate via a DNA intermediate. The diploid RNA genome is transcribed after infection into a single molecule of DNA by the enzyme reverse transcriptase, present in the virion. This DNA circularises and is integrated into the cellular genome after entering the nucleus. Both viral messenger RNA and virion RNA are then transcribed from this integrated provirus by cellular enzymes. Nucleocapsids are assembled in the cytoplasm and acquire their envelope by budding through the cell membrane. This multiplication process is often compatible with cell survival, although it may affect cell function and/or metabolism. The basic structure of the retrovirus genome is shown in Figure 6.2, although this is subject to much variation in individual viruses.

The integrated provirus is essentially equivalent to a cellular gene, although it is controlled by its own promoter. The complete infectious cycle is undergone by exogenous retroviruses such as human immunodeficiency virus or human T-cell lymphotropic virus (HTLV). When such viruses infect the germ line, however, retroviral insertions into the chromosome can acquire the status of permanent genes, and be transmitted to progeny. In fact this has occurred many times during human evolution, so that such sequences represent about 8% of the human genome. This gene category is as yet poorly studied and understood (44).

Association with MS

Among the first reports of the association of retroviruses with MS was the finding that some MS patients respond immunologically to a retrovirus that is related to HTLV. This virus was also present in cerebrospinal T cells from MS patients. This report was based largely on immunological evidence from enzyme-linked immunosorbent assays with viral antigens (45). However, a later study failed to confirm these findings (46).

A retrovirus was again associated with MS patients in a subsequent study (44), but this was a different retrovirus which was characterised at the molecular level and was unrelated to HTLV. This virus was termed MS-associated retrovirus (MSRV), and was repeatedly isolated from leptomeningeal, choroids plexus, and EBV-immortalized B cells of MS patients. Retrovirus sequences were detected by polymerase chain reaction from sucrose gradient purified extracellular virions. The same sequence was detected in the plasma, cerebrospinal fluid, peripheral blood mononuclear cells, and brain of MS patients (47, 48). Sequence analysis showed that this virus was related to an endogenous retrovirus sequence which is now known to be a family of human endogenous retrovirus (HERV) elements, named HERV-W (49). Numerous studies have now suggested that MSRV expression is associated with the epidemiology, clinical progression, and prognosis of MS (44).

MSRV ENV protein has been shown to be a potent immunogen. It induces activation of innate immunity and release of proinflammatory cytokines such as interferon-γ, through toll-like receptor 4 agonist effect (50). The association with MS is emphasised by the detection of ENV protein and RNA in demyelinated tissue in autopsy samples from MS patients. In one study, quantitative RT-PCR with primers specific for MSRV/HERV-W ENV and POL was used to determine virus copy numbers. Brain sections were immuno-stained with HERV-W ENV-specific monoclonal antibody to detect the viral protein. All brains expressed MSRV/HERV-W ENV and POL genes. Accumulation of MSRV/HERV-W-specific RNAs was greater in MS brains than in controls. By immunohistochemistry, no HERV-W ENV protein was detected in control brains, whereas it was up-regulated within MS plaques and correlated with the extent of active demyelination and inflammation (48). In a separate study, antigen expression of HERV-W, in normal human brain and MS lesions, was studied by immunohistochemistry. A panel of antibodies against ENV and GAG antigens was tested. A physiological expression of GAG proteins in neuronal cells was observed in normal brain, whereas there was a striking accumulation of GAG antigen in axonal structures in demyelinated white matter from patients with MS. Prominent HERV-W GAG expression was also detected in endothelial cells of MS lesions from acute or actively demyelinating cases, a pattern not found in any control. A physiological expression of ENV proteins was detected in microglia in normal brain; however, a specific expression in macrophages was restricted to early MS lesions. Thus GAG and ENV proteins encoded by the HERV-W are expressed in cells of the CNS under normal conditions and HERV-W GAG may thus have a physiological function in human brain. This expression differs in MS lesions, which is compatible with a pathophysiological role in MS, but also illustrates that HERV antigens can be expressed in cell-specific patterns, under physiological or patho-logical conditions, in normal or MS brain (51).

MSRV has also been associated with a more severe prognosis, in that patients showing MSRV in the CSF using nested PCR for the POL gene showed a greater number of relapses and entry into the progressive phase than those negative for MSRV (52). This has been attributed to the gliotoxic properties of MSRV (53).

Natalizumab and progressive multifocal leukoencephalopathy

Natalizumab is a humanised monoclonal antibody that was developed by Elan Pharma-ceuticals and Biogen Idec for the treatment of relapsing–remitting MS. It has the trade name Tysabri and was formerly called Antegren (54).

In MS, inflammatory CNS lesions arise from the migration of activated lymphocytes and monocytes across the vascular endothelium of the CNS. These cells express the glycoprotein $\alpha_4$integrin on their surface, which plays an essential role in their adhesion to the vascular endothelium and migration into the parenchyma. Natalizumab is an

$\alpha_4$integrin antagonist which reduces migration of such cells and hence the development of inflammatory CNS lesions (55).

Natalizumab is given by intravenous infusion monthly. In one randomized, double-blind clinical trial, 213 patients with relapsing–remitting or relapsing secondary progressive MS were given natalizumab or a placebo. There was a marked reduction in the number of new lesions in the natalizumab treated groups, as measured by magnetic resonance imaging, as well as in the number of relapses (55). This and other clinical trials have shown that natalizumab is both well tolerated and effective.

The most important adverse effect of natalizumab is the occurrence of progressive multifocal leukoencephalopathy (PML), a usually fatal degenerative disease of the CNS. In initial clinical trials of the drug there were three cases of PML: two in patients with MS on combination therapy with intramuscular interferon beta-1a and one in a patient with Crohn's disease (an inflammatory disease of the gut) who had been treated with various immunosuppressants and immunomodulators. Examination of 3116 patients enrolled in clinical trials indicated a risk of developing PML of about 1 in 1000 cases after a mean of 18 monthly doses. Natalizumab was approved by the US Food and Drug Administration in 2004 (56), but was subsequently withdrawn from the market by the manufacturers after it was linked with PML. A safety evaluation was carried out, and the drug returned to the market in 2006 after there were no more fatalities. However, up to October 2009 there have been 24 cases of PML worldwide in patients given natalizumab. It is now recommended for use for severe cases of relapsing–remitting MS, and only as a monotherapy, since cases of PML initially appeared to be linked to the use of other medications (57).

JC virus

JC virus is the etiological agent of PML, named from the initials of the patient in whom it was first discovered. It is a human polyomavirus with a small supercoiled and circular DNA genome and an icosahedral capsid (58). The cellular receptor for JCV on glial cells is a serotonin receptor. It causes usually asymptomatic infections of children and approximately 80% of the adult population are seropositive. The virus remains latent after primary infection but the form that the latency takes is not known. PML occurs largely in people with AIDS and other forms of immune impairment (59).

There is controversy over whether natalizumab can induce increased JC virus expression in MS patients who do not have PML. One study described an increased prevalence of JC virus DNA in 19 patients with MS after 12 to 18 months of treatment with natalizumab (60). These findings contrast with results from other groups (61).

Progressive multifocal leukoencephalopathy

PML is a demyelinating disease of the CNS, caused by JC virus infection. Before the AIDS epidemic, PML was a rare disease in immunosuppressed patients, for example those with lymphoma and leukaemia. PML now occurs mostly in AIDS patients, and 5% of such patients develop PML (59, 62). The clinical signs of PML are impaired speech and vision, dementia or confusion, and varying degrees of paralysis. Subsequent disease progression is rapid, with clinical signs intensifying and death of the patient usually occurring within 3 to 6 months (59).

PML is a lytic infection of oligodendrocytes and is characterised by enlarged oligo-dendrocytes with nuclear inclusion bodies and crystalline arrays of viral particles. This results in lesions which occur in the cerebrum, cerebellum, and brain stem. Astrocytes are infected non-permissively, whereas neurons are not infected; however, B cells and mono-nuclear cells are infected (63), and it is possible that lymphocytes act as a reservoir and dissemination vehicle (64).

MS and PML are demyelinating diseases of the CNS, but they can be distinguished at the histopathological level by the inclusion bodies within the nuclei of oligodendroctyes and the lack of inflammatory infiltrates, which are characteristic of PML (65). However, the similarity between MS and PML has led to investigations of the association between JC re-activation and MS, with contradictory results. Some studies have found JC virus DNA in the CSF of some MS patients but not in controls (66), whereas others have found no evidence for JC virus re-activation in MS patients (67).

Risk assessment

The risk of developing PML increases with the number of natalizumab infusions received. At present, the US Food and Drug Administration Tysabri risk management plan, called the TOUCH Prescribing Program, gives guidelines for the prescription of natalizumab (68). TOUCH stands for Tysabri Outreach: Unified Commitment to Health. It is a restricted distribution programme which allows only prescribers and patients enrolled in the programme to prescribe and receive natalizumab. Its aim is to balance risk against patient benefit. In the European Union natalizumab is indicated as a single disease modifying therapy in highly active relapsing–remitting MS, for patients with high disease activity despite treatment with a beta-interferon, or in patients with rapidly evolving severe relapsing–remitting MS (69).

Human viruses and MS

The basic hypothesis underlying the etiology of MS, namely that an environmental factor triggers the disease at around the age of adolescence, and this is manifested later as disease symptoms, has not changed for the last 20 years. The other long-lasting hypothesis is that the disease is related to an interaction between environmental factor(s) and genetic factors. The idea that a virus could be an environmental factor also has a long history, but here the evidence is variable and often contradictory, and much controversy has surrounded this idea. In this chapter evidence relating to the involvement of measles, rubella, herpes (of five types), and retroviruses has been discussed.

The idea that a virus infection around the age of adolescence could trigger MS is an attractive one, and two scenarios could be envisaged. The first is that MS is associated with an ongoing or persistent infection that continuously triggers the inflammatory demyelination. The second is that the virus infection is 'hit and run', that is that the virus infects, and then disappears, but triggers a disease process that eventually manifests itself as overt MS.

Searches for the presence of viral 'footprints', that is the virus itself or viral nucleic acid, have been made for the viruses implicated in MS, and also immunity against these viruses in MS patients has been measured. In all cases the presence of viral footprints is claimed in only a proportion of MS cases, and this is also true of raised immunity. Therefore, it can never be claimed that a single virus is implicated in the etiology of MS.

It is clear from studies of the neuropathology of MS that it is a heterogeneous disease. For example, different patterns of demyelination can be distinguished, including demyelination with relative preservation of oligodendrocytes, myelin destruction with concomitant and complete destruction of oligodendrocytes, or primary destruction or disturbance of myelinating cells with secondary demyelination (70). In some cases a primary demyelination may be followed by a secondary oligodendrocyte loss in the established lesions. Some severe conditions may result in destructive lesions with loss of myelin, oligodendrocytes, axons, and astrocytes. Thus generally four distinct patterns of demyelination may be differentiated (71). This heterogeneity of pathology may mean that different immunological pathways may lead to the formation of plaques, indicating that the demyelinated plaques of MS may reflect a common pathological end point of different pathological mechanisms.

This heterogeneity in MS lesions, combined with differences in the clinical course of the disease and its response to treatment, may in turn reflect the fact that there may be several etiological mechanisms in MS, and not just one. Given these facts, the search for a single viral cause of MS may be futile. Indeed there may also be non-viral factors in the etiology of MS, including perhaps sunlight and vitamin D (72).

One of the problems with claims for the presence of viruses in MS tissue is that it is more difficult to publish negative than positive data. However, one study has searched for the presence of six different neurotropic viruses, including JC virus (JCV), VZV, HHV-6, and EBV, in CSF samples collected from 51 patients with MS and 30 patients with other neurological diseases (73). Cell-free or cell-associated viral DNA in CSF samples was detected by real-time PCR, and viral loads were determined. Magnetic resonance imaging examinations were also performed to look for active lesions. Cell-associated JCV DNA was detected in 3 of the 51 patients with MS and in 2 of the 30 patients with other neurological disease. Cell-free JCV DNA was detected in one additional patient with MS. Cell-free VZV DNA was detected in one patient without MS, cell-free HHV-6 was detected in one patient with MS, and cell-free EBV was detected in one patient with MS. All other study patients had no detectable viral DNA in CSF samples and no double infections were found. The small percentage of patients with detectable viral DNA in CSF samples was comparable between patients with MS and those with other neurological disease, and presence of viral DNA was not a predictor of brain lesions. Therefore, in this study the large majority of MS patients do not show the presence of the viruses sought and there is no correlation with brain lesions.

That viruses may induce CNS demyelination after infectious virus has been cleared has been shown by studies of two mouse model systems, Semliki Forest virus and JHM coronavirus, although the time period involved is short (see Chapter 5). For Theiler's virus, demyelination is linked to virus persistence. However, it is at least possible that a virus may act as a trigger for CNS demyelination and does not need to be present in infectious form.

The hypothesis that a virus or viruses may be involved in the etiology of MS remains unproven, although several candidates have emerged, as described in previous chapters. If a virus is involved in MS, it seems most likely that the virus infection acts as a trigger and that virus persistence, if it occurs, may be irrelevant (74). It may be that the initial stimulation of anti-myelin immunity may be triggered by a virus, either by direct infection of the CNS or by molecular mimicry, but this may not be a unique property of a single virus. It is possible that this initial autoimmunity may be magnified by immune-mediated damage and epitope spreading, until the symptoms of MS appear many years later.

This is but one hypothesis out of several that have been advanced to explain the etiology of MS. However, the mechanisms of triggering of MS and of progression of the disease remain mysteries despite many years of experimentation and deliberation.

References

1. Sips, G.J., Chesik, D., Glazenburg, L., Wilschut, J., and De Jeyser, J. (2007). Involvement of morbilliviruses in the pathogenesis of demyelinating disease. *Rev. Med. Virol.* **17**, 223–244.

2. Frey, T.K. (1997). Neurological aspects of rubella virus infection. *Intervirology* **40**, 167–175.

3. Bachmann, S. and Kesselring, J. (1998). Multiple sclerosis and infectious childhood diseases. *Neuroepidemiology* **17**, 154–160.

4. Bager, P., Nielsen, N.M., Bihrmann, K., *et al.* (2004). Childhood infections and risk of multiple sclerosis. *Brain* **127**, 2491–2497.

5. Kerdiles, Y.M., Sellin, C.I., Druelle, J., and Horvat, B. (2006). Immunosuppression caused by measles virus: role of viral proteins. *Rev. Med. Virol.* **16**, 49–63.

6. Edlich, R.F., Winters, K.L., Long, W.B. 3rd, and Gubler, K.D. (2005). Rubella and congenital rubella (German measles). *J. Long Term Eff. Med. Implants* **15**, 319–328.

7. Chantler, J., Wolinsky, J., and Tingle, A. (2001). Rubella virus. In: *Fields Virology*, 4th Ed.; Knipe, D.M. and Howley, P.M., Eds. Lippincott, Williams and Wilkins, Philadelphia, 963–990.

8. Menge, T., Kieseier, B.C., Nessler, S., Hemmer, B., Hartung, H.P., and Stüve, O. (2007). Acute disseminated encephalomyelitis: an acute hit against the brain. *Curr. Opin. Neurol.* **20**, 247–254.

9. Rima, B.K. and Duprex, W.P. (2006). Morbilliviruses and human disease. *J. Pathol.* **208**, 199–214.

10. Smith-Jensen, T., Burgoon, M.P., Anthony, J., Kraus, H., Gilden, D.H., and Owens, G.P. (2000). Comparison of immunoglobulin G heavy-chain sequences in MS and SSPE brains reveals an antigen-driven response. *Neurology* **54**, 1227–1232.

11. Ter Meulen, V. and Hall, W.W. (1978). Slow virus infections of the nervous system: virological, immunological and pathogenetic considerations. *J. Gen. Virol.* **41**, 1–25.

12. Pohl-Koppe, A., Kaiser, R., Meulen, V.T., and Liebert, U.G. (1995). Antibody reactivity to individual structural proteins of measles virus in the CSF of SSPE and MS patients. *Clin. Diagn. Virol.* **4**, 135–147.

13. Nath, A. and Wolinsky, J.S. (1990). Antibody response to rubella virus structural proteins in multiple sclerosis. *Ann. Neurol.* **27**, 533–536.

14. Rohowsky-Kochan, C., Dowling, P.C., and Cook, S.D. (1995). Canine distemper virus-specific antibodies in multiple sclerosis. *Neurology* **45**, 1554–1560.

15. Jarius, S., Eichhorn, P., Jacobi, C., Wildemann, B., Wick, M., and Voltz, R. (2009). The intrathecal, polyspecific antiviral immune response: specific for MS or a general marker of CNS autoimmunity? *J. Neurol. Sci.* **280**, 98–100.

16. Cosby, S.L., McQuaid, S., Taylor, M.J., *et al.* (1989). Examination of eight cases of multiple sclerosis and 56 neurological and non-neurological controls for genomic sequences of measles virus, canine distemper virus, simian virus 5 and rubella virus. *J. Gen. Virol.* **70**, 2027–2036.

17. Brankin, B., Osman, M., Herlihy, L., Hawkins, S.A., and Cosby, S.L. (1996). Failure to detect measles virus RNA, by reverse transcription-polymerase chain reaction, in peripheral blood leucocytes of patients with multiple sclerosis. *Mult. Scler.* **1**, 204–206.

18. Ahlgren, C., Odén, A., Torén, K., and Andersen O. (2009). Multiple sclerosis incidence in the era of measles-mumps-rubella mass vaccinations. *Acta Neurol. Scand.* **119**, 313–320.

19. Atkins, G.J., McQuaid, S., Morris-Downes, M.M., et al. (2000). Transient virus infection and multiple sclerosis. *Rev. Med. Virol.* **10**, 291–303.

20. Lucchinetti, C.F., Brück, W., Rodriguez, M., and Lassmann, H. (1996). Distinct patterns of multiple sclerosis pathology indicates heterogeneity on pathogenesis. *Brain Pathol.* **6**, 259–274.

21. Simmons, A. (2001). Herpesviruses and multiple sclerosis. *Herpes* **8**, 60–63.

22. McHatters, G.R. and Scham, R.G. (1995). Bird viruses and multiple sclerosis: combination of viruses or Marek's alone? *Neurosci. Lett.* **188**, 75–76.

23. Roizman, B. and Pellett, P.E. (2001). The family Herpesviridae: a brief introduction. In: *Fields Virology*, 4th Ed.; Knipe, D.M. and Howley, P.M., Eds. Lippincott, Williams and Wilkins, Philadelphia, 2381–2399.

24. Martin, J.R. (1981). Herpes simplex virus types 1 and 2 in multiple sclerosis. *Lancet* **2**, 777–781.

25. Ferrante, P., Mancuso, R., Pagani, E., et al. (2000). Molecular evidences for a role of HSV-1 in multiple sclerosis clinical acute attack. *J. Neurovirol.* **6 (Suppl 2)**, S109–114.

26. Jarius, S., Eichhorn, P., Jacobi, C., Wildemann, B., Wick, M., and Voltz, R. (2009). The intrathecal, polyspecific antiviral immune response: specific for MS or a general marker of CNS autoimmunity? *J. Neurol. Sci.* **280**, 98–100.

27. Mancuso, R., Delbue, S., Borghi, E., et al. (2007). Increased prevalence of varicella zoster virus DNA in cerebrospinal fluid from patients with multiple sclerosis. *J. Med. Virol.* **79**, 192–199.

28. Sotelo, J., Martinez-Palomo, A., Ordofiez, G., and Pineda, B. (2008). Varicella-zoster virus in cerebrospinal fluid at relapses of multiple sclerosis. *Ann. Neurol.* **63**, 303–311.

29. Gilden, D.H. (2008). Is varicella zoster virus really involved in the pathogenesis of multiple sclerosis? *Ann. Neurol.* **63**, 269–271.

30. Burgoon, M.P., Cohrs, R.J., Bennett, J.L., et al. (2009). Varicella zoster virus is not a disease-relevant antigen in multiple sclerosis. *Ann. Neurol.* **65**, 474–479.

31. Fotheringham, J. and Jacobson, S. (2005). Human herpesvirus 6 and multiple sclerosis: potential mechanisms for virus-induced disease. *Herpes* **12**, 4–9.

32. Cermelli, C., Berti, R., Soldan, S.S., et al. (2003). High frequency of human herpesvirus 6 DNA in multiple sclerosis plaques isolated by laser microdissection. *J. Infect. Dis.* **187**, 1377–1387.

33. Mameli, G., Astone, V., Arru, G., et al. (2007). Brains and peripheral blood mononuclear cells of multiple sclerosis (MS) patients hyperexpress MS-associated retrovirus/HERV-W endogenous retrovirus, but not human herpesvirus 6. *J. Gen. Virol.* **88**, 264–274.

34. Cirone, M., Cuomo, L., Zompetta, C., et al. (2002). Human herpesvirus 6 and multiple sclerosis: a study of T cell cross-reactivity to viral and myelin basic protein antigens. *J. Med. Virol.* **68**, 268–272.

35. Tejada-Simon, M.V., Zang, Y.C., Hong, J., Riviera, V.M., and Zang, J.Z. (2003). Cross-reactivity with myelin basic protein and human herpesvirus-6 in multiple sclerosis. *Ann. Neurol.* **53**, 189–197.

36. Pohl, D. (2009). Epstein-Barr virus and multiple sclerosis. *J. Neurol. Sci.* **286**, 62–64.

37. Thacker, E.L., Mirzael, F., and Ascherio, A. (2006). Infectious mononucleosis and risk for multiple sclerosis: a meta-analysis. *Ann. Neurol.* **59**, 499–503.

38. Serafini, B., Rosicarelli, B., Franciotta, D., et al. (2007). Dysregulated Epstein-Barr virus infection in the multiple sclerosis brain. *J. Exp. Med.* **204**, 2899–2912.

39. Willis, S.N., Stadelmann, C., Rodig, S.J., et al. (2009). Epstein-Barr virus infection is not a characteristic feature of multiple sclerosis brain. *Brain* **132**, 3318–3328.

40. Peferoen, L.A.N., Lamers, F., Lenthe, N.R., et al. (2010). Epstein-Barr virus is not a characteristic feature in the central nervous system in established multiple sclerosis. *Brain* **133**, 1–4.

41. Reiber, H. and Peter, J.B. (2001). Cerebrospinal fluid analysis: disease-related data patterns and evaluation programs. *J. Neurol. Sci.* **184**, 101–122.

42. Lünemann, J.D., Edwards, N., Muraro, P.A., *et al.* (2006). Increased frequency and broadened specificity of latent EBV nuclear antigen-1-specific T cells in multiple sclerosis. *Brain* **129**, 1493–1506.

43. Lünemann, J.D., Jelcić, I., Roberts, S., *et al.* (2008). EBNA1-specific T cells from patients with multiple sclerosis cross react with myelin antigens and co-produce IFN-gamma and IL-2. *J. Exp. Med.* **205**, 1763–1773.

44. Perron, H., Berbard, C., Bertrand, J.-B., *et al.* (2009). Endogenous retroviral genes, herpesviruses and gender in multiple sclerosis. *J. Neurol. Sci.* **286**, 65–72.

45. Koprowski, H., DeFreitas, E.C., Harper, M.E., *et al.* (1985). Multiple sclerosis and human T-cell lymphotropic retroviruses. *Nature* **318**, 154–160.

46. Karpas, A., Kämpf, U., Sidèn, A., Koch, M., and Poser, S. (1986). Lack of evidence for involvement of known human retroviruses in multiple sclerosis. *Nature* **322**, 177–178.

47. Perron, H., Garson, J.A., Bedin, F., *et al.* (1997). Molecular identification of a novel retrovirus repeatedly isolated from patients with multiple sclerosis. *Proc. Natl. Acad. Sci. U.S.A.* **94**, 7583–7588.

48. Mameli, G., Astone, V., Arru, G., *et al.* (2007). Brains and peripheral blood mononuclear cells of multiple sclerosis (MS) patients hyperexpress MS-associated retrovirus/HERV-W endogenous retrovirus, but not human herpesvirus 6. *J. Gen. Virol.* **88**, 264–274.

49. Blond, J.L., Besème, F., Duret, L., *et al.* (1999). Molecular characterization and placental expression of HERV-W, a new human endogenous retrovirus family. *J. Virol.* **73**, 1175–1185.

50. Rolland, A., Jouvin-Marche, E., Viret, C., Faure, M., Perron, H., and Marche, P.N. (2006). The envelope protein of a human endogenous retrovirus-W family activates innate immunity through CD14/TLR-4 and promotes Th1-like responses. *J. Immunol.* **176**, 7636–7644.

51. Perron, H., Lazarini, F., Ruprecht, K., *et al.* (2005). Human endogenous retrovirus (HERV)-W ENV and GAG proteins: physiological expression in human brain and pathophysiological modulation in multiple sclerosis lesions. *J. Neurovirol.* **11**, 23–33.

52. Sotgiu, S., Serra, C., Mameli, G., *et al.* (2006). Multiple sclerosis-associated retrovirus in early multiple sclerosis: a six-year follow-up of a Sardinian cohort. *Mult. Scler.* **12**, 698–703.

53. Sotgiu, S., Serra, C., Mameli, G., *et al.* (2002). Multiple sclerosis-associated retrovirus and MS prognosis: an observational study. *Neurology* **59**, 1071–1073.

54. Natalizumab. Wikopedia. http://en.wikipedia.org/wiki/Natalizumab

55. Miller, D.H., Khan, O.A., Sheremata, W.A., *et al.* (2003). A controlled trial of natalizumab for relapsing multiple sclerosis. *New Engl. J. Med.* **348**, 15–23.

56. Natalizumab (marketed as Tysabri). US Food and Drug Administration. http://www.fda.gov/Safety/MedWatch/SafetyInformation/SafetyAlertsforHumanMedicalProducts/ucm182667.htm

57. UPDATE 1-EU agency reports 24th case of Tysabri infection. Reuters. http://www.reuters.com/article/idUSLT39797520091029

58. Major, E.O. (2001). Human polyomavirus. In: *Fields Virology*, 4th Ed.; Knipe, D.M. and Howley, P.M., Eds. Lippincott, Williams and Wilkins, Philadelphia, 2175–2196.

59. Mengxi, J.I., Abend, J.R., Johnson, S.F., and Imperiale, M.J. (2009). The role of polyomaviruses in human disease. *Virology* **384**, 266–273.

60. Chen, Y., Bord, E., Tompkins, T., *et al.* (2009). Asymptomatic reactivation of JC virus in patients treated with natalizumab. *New Engl. J. Med.* **361**, 1067–1074.

61. Gorelik, L., Goelz, S., and Sandrock, A.W. (2009). Asymptomatic reactivation of JC virus in patients treated with natalizumab (letter). *New Engl. J. Med.* **361**, 2487–2488.

62. Berger, J.R. (2003). Progressive multifocal leukoencephalopathy in acquired immunodeficiency syndrome: explaining the high incidence and disproportionate frequency of the illness relative to other immunosuppressive conditions. *J. Neurovirol.* **9 (Suppl 1)**, 38–41.

63. von Einsiedel, R.W., Samorei, I.W., Pawlita, M., Zwissler, B., Deubel, M., and Vinters, H.V. (2004). New JC virus infection patterns by in situ polymerase chain reaction in brains of acquired immunodeficiency syndrome patients with progressive multifocal leukoencephalopathy. *J. Neurovirol.* **10**, 1–11.

64. Doerries, K., Sbiera, S., Drews, K., Arendt, G., Eggers, C., and Doerries, R. (2003). Association of human polyomavirus JC with peripheral blood of immunoimpaired and healthy individuals. *J. Neurovirol.* **9 (Suppl 1)**, 81–87.

65. Khalili, K., White, M.K., Lublin, F., Ferrante, P., and Berger, J.R. (2007). Reactivation of JC virus and development of PML in patients with multiple sclerosis. *Neurology* **68**, 985–990.

66. Ferrante, P., Omodeo-Zorini, E., Caldarelli-Stefano, R., *et al.* (1998). Detection of JC virus DNA in cerebrospinal fluid from multiple sclerosis patients. *Mult. Scler.* **4**, 49–54.

67. Bogdanovic, G., Priftakis, P., Hammarin, A.L., *et al.* (1998). Detection of JC virus in cerebrospinal fluid (CSF) samples from patients with progressive multifocal leukoencephalopathy but not in CSF samples from patients with herpes simplex encephalitis, enteroviral meningitis, or multiple sclerosis. *J. Clin. Microbiol.* **36**, 1137–1138.

68. Tysabri® (natalizumab): TOUCH Prescribing Program. http://www.tysabri.com/safety-with-tysabri.xml

69. Tysabri approved for return in Europe. http://www.thisisms.com/article274.html

70. Lucchinetti, C.F., Brück, W., Rodriguez, M., and Lassmann, H. (1996). Distinct patterns of multiple sclerosis pathology indicates heterogeneity on pathogenesis. *Brain Pathol.* **6**, 259–274.

71. Kornek, B. and Lassmann, H. (2003). Neuropathology of multiple sclerosis: new concepts. *Brain Res. Bull.* **61**, 321–326.

72. Ascherio, A., Munger, K.L., and Simon, K.C. (2010). Vitamin D and multiple sclerosis. *Lancet Neurol.* **9**, 599–612.

73. Mancuso, R., Hernis, A., Cavarretta, R., *et al.* (2010). Detection of viral DNA sequences in the cerebrospinal fluid of patients with multiple sclerosis. *J. Med. Virol.* **82**, 1051–1057.

74. Atkins, G.J., McQuaid, S., Morris-Downes, M.M., *et al.* (2000). Transient virus infection and multiple sclerosis. *Rev. Med. Virol.* **10**, 291–303.

Epilogue: conclusions and future directions

7

Gregory J. Atkins, Kingston H.G. Mills, Paul van der Valk
and Sandra Amor

A large amount of scientific and clinical research has been carried out on MS. This has
been aimed at understanding the pathogenesis of the disease and at developing new
treatment strategies. We now have a large amount of information concerning MS
pathogenesis and the mechanisms are becoming elucidated, both for the disease itself
and for EAE and viral models. A main tenet of MS research, first put forward by Dean
and colleagues (1), is that MS is triggered by an environmental factor that exerts its
effects around adolescence, in genetically susceptible individuals. This general mechanism is still accepted. However, the difficulty comes when these interacting factors are
further dissected.

Many animal and human diseases are characterised by CNS demyelination, therefore it
has been assumed that a likely candidate for the environmental factor postulated in MS is a
virus. This has prompted a search for viruses associated with MS. However, this search has
led to equivocal results and no one virus has been definitely associated with MS. It may be
that several viruses may be responsible, since MS is a disease of varying pathologies (2), each
of which may be associated with a different etiology. There may also be an interaction
between viruses and other environmental factors, for example activation of herpes viruses
caused by vitamin D deficiency (3). The second problem which may be associated with the
virus hypothesis is that the virus may not persist in MS tissue, but may be associated with a
'hit and run' mechanism, so a later search for the virus may be fruitless (4). Also a problem
here is that it is more difficult to publish negative rather than positive claims, so the
literature contains many claims for etiological agents associated with MS, not many of
which have been refuted or confirmed.

In terms of animal models for MS, EAE is the most realistic. However, it is difficult to
envisage how the induction of EAE could be triggered naturally, except perhaps by myelin
damage, which could in turn be caused by a virus. The three main viral models of MS have
drawbacks. The Theiler's virus model involves virus persistence, and so may not represent a
realistic model for MS, although the mechanisms of demyelination are like MS. The Semliki
Forest virus and JHM coronavirus models show transient demyelination over the short
term, although virus does not persist. Thus there is also a problem with these models in
comparing to MS. The best viral animal model would be one where long-term chronic
demyelination (similar to chronic EAE) is triggered by a virus infection but where the virus
does not persist. However, such a model does not yet exist.

The other environmental factor that has been implicated in MS is vitamin D and UV irradiation. However, as with viruses, the results have been equivocal. This idea certainly correlates with the increase in MS frequency with latitude. However, a large study of vitamin D levels and MS incidence is required before any conclusions can be drawn. Randomised controlled clinical trials are the next step in addressing whether vitamin D prevents MS or can favourably affect the course and progression of MS (5).

Studies have indicated that the genetic control of MS is complex and polygenic, but the genes associated with T cell-mediated immunity are prevalent. The latest study has involved collaboration between several institutes (6). Thus it is unlikely that a simple explanation for the inheritance of MS susceptibility will be advanced and more work will probably contribute to the large number of genes already known to influence MS susceptibility.

Significant progress has been made in the last few years in our understanding of the pathogenesis of MS, based on studies in MS patients and in EAE. While it has long been accepted that T cells, as well as B cells and innate immune responses, play a major role in loss of tolerance to self antigens, there has been a paradigm shift following the discovery of Th17 cells, and their acceptance as a distinct population from Th1 cells that are primarily responsible for disease pathology in many autoimmune diseases. Indeed much of the effort in drug development for T cell-mediated autoimmune diseases is now focused around blocking Th17 cells, their induction, migration, or function.

It was initially thought that IFN-γ-secreting Th1 cells mediate pathology in the CNS of MS patients. However, mice deficient in IFN-γ or IFN-γ receptors had increased susceptibility to EAE (7) and treatment of mice with IFN-γ protected against EAE (8). Furthermore, mice defective in IL-12 (IL-12p35$^{-/-}$ mice) had exacerbated disease (9). In contrast, mice defective in IL-23, a critical cytokine involved in induction of expansion of Th17 cells, or mice deficient in IL-17 had reduced susceptibility to EAE (9, 10). Furthermore, EAE could be induced by transfer of myelin-specific Th17 from mice with EAE (11). Consistent with these studies in mice, IL-17 mRNA was found to be elevated in the CSF and blood of patients with MS (12). Furthermore CD4+ T cells from MS patients have enhanced IL-17 production and DCs have enhanced IL-23 production, when compared with corresponding cells from healthy individuals (13).

The development and expansion of Th17 cells is controlled by complex combinations of cytokines. Although IL-23 was the first to be discovered, it now appears that it may not be the critical differentiation factor for Th17 cells, but is required in co-operation with other cytokines, such as IL-1 or IL-18 for expansion of Th17 cell, and for promoting innate IL-17 production by $\gamma\delta$ T cells (14–18). In contrast, IL-6, IL-21, and TGF-β have been implicated in the differentiation of Th17 cells (19, 20). Antibodies and inhibitors of IL-6, IL-1, IL-21, and IL-23 are each being accessed as therapeutics against in a variety of autoimmune diseases. An antibody against IL-12p40, ustekinumab, which blocks the function of IL-12 and IL-23, has considerable clinical efficacy against psoriasis, psoriatic arthritis, and Crohn's disease and has already been licensed for psoriasis (21). Although IL-12p40$^{-/-}$ mice are resistant to EAE and treatment with antibodies to IL-12p40 reduced the clinical symptoms of EAE (22), ustekinumab failed to reduce the number of brain lesions in patients with relapsing–remitting MS (23). There are a number of explanations for this, including the possibility that IL-23 functions more in the precipitation of autoimmune inflammation rather than in disease relapse or needs to gain access to the CNS for activation of local Th17 cells, or indeed that EAE is not a good model for MS. Nevertheless, these findings do not rule out a role for IL-23, IL-17, or Th17 in the pathology of MS, but suggests that more research is required to fully understand the factors that provoke and re-activate the pathogenic T cells that mediate inflammation in MS and how these can be exploited to develop more effective therapies.

The current first-line immunomodulatory therapies for MS, IFN-β and glatiramer acetate, are only modestly effective and only work in a proportion of patients. Non-responder patients are often treated with natalizumab (Tysabri), an anti-VLA-4 antibody that inhibits leucocyte traffic across the blood–brain barrier. Although natilizumab is effective in patients with relapsing MS who do not respond to IFN-β1a (24), it is associated with a risk of developing potentially fatal progressive multifocal leukoencephalopathy (PML) (25). However this risk may be reduced by screening patients for the virus that provokes PML. An alternative approach for inhibiting migration of encephalogenic T cells has involved preventing lymphocyte egress from lymph nodes using a sphingosine-1-phosphate (S1P) inhibitor, FTY720 (fingolimod). This has the advantage over other therapies of being the first orally effective drug for treating MS. An alternative approach has involved depleting T cells, B cells, and monocytes with an anti-CD52 antibody (Alemtuzumab) and this has been shown to be more effective than IFN-β in clinical trials involving patients with relapsing–remitting MS (26).

Although rationally designed immunomodulatory therapies are a step up from the more traditional drugs for the treatment of MS, these drugs still do not specifically target the pathogenic immune cells and future research on the mechanisms of immune-mediated pathology has the capacity to deliver more effective drugs. For example, there is considerable evidence from mouse models that the IL-1 family of cytokines plays a key role in driving Th17 responses in mouse models of autoimmune inflammation. Although there are no reports of success with IL-1 targeted therapies in MS, studies in the EAE model have shown redundancy between cytokines processed by caspase-1 and the inflammasome in promoting IL-17 production in synergy with IL-23 (18). Therefore blocking IL-1β and IL-18 using small molecule inhibitors of the inflammasome may be more effective than blocking IL-1 alone. Apart from the problems of targeting the cell in the appropriate tissue at the appropriate stage of the disease, another major issue faced by approaches that non-specifically block lymphocyte migration or induction of discrete T cell subtypes is that of compromising host immunity. Patients on anti-inflammatory biologics, including drugs that target TNFα (infliximab) (27), IL-12p40 (ustekinumab) (18), or VLA-4 (natalizumab) (25) can be more susceptible to certain infections and cancers.

Strategies designed to stimulate the patient's own anti-inflammatory mediators, such as IL-10, TGF-β, or IL-27, may have greater specificity with reduced risks of infection. It has recently been shown that the high frequency of patients that fail to respond to IFN-β do not produce IL-27 (28) and it was suggested that IL-27 or agents that induce its production in vivo may be more effective than IFN-β in treating MS. Alternatively, studies in mice have shown that it may be possible to treat MS patients by inducing or transfusing regulatory T (Treg) cells specific for autoantigens, such as myelin basic protein (MBP), which is believed to be the target for pathogenic T cells in MS. Transfer of MBP-specific Treg cells is effective against disease induction and progression in the EAE model (29). These approaches have the advantage of confining the suppression to the site of antigen expression and inflammation and may reduce the issues associated with drugs that broadly suppress immune responses and compromise host immunity to infection.

It has long since been accepted that MS is an autoimmune disease in which the target is myelin, a complex structure containing at least some sequestered antigens. Damage to the myelin could elicit an immune response leading to additional damage which would then result in a vicious circle consisting of progressive attacks. This 'determinant spreading' has been proposed to underlay the chronicity of MS. In animal models this does not always, if at all, seem to be the case. Moreover, damage to the brain, as in stroke for example, does not lead to MS.

In MS, bouts of remyelination follow lesion formation, leading to the typical relapsing–remitting course of damage/repair in the brain and the clinical symptoms. Evidence cited for this sequence of events is the presence of autoantibodies and autoreactive T cells, some response to immunosuppressive drugs (at least at the start of the disease), and the similarities to an autoimmune disease model (EAE).

As discussed in Chapter 3 classical EAE involving immunisation with myelin or myelin proteins induces inflammation and some demyelination, but this acute model is a self-limiting disease in which the pathology does not resemble chronic MS. Manipulation of the model (selection of different strains/animals, feeding the animals cyclosporine, use of adjuvants, for example) can make the pathology look more like MS. However, it is probably not a good model for MS, though it can be very useful to follow the different processes that are seen in MS.

Questions over the validity of the autoimmune hypothesis for MS have come from several different findings. Most important is the fact that most of the immunosuppressive regimens currently used for treating MS are partially effective in the early years of the disease, after which the efficacy decreases. Though the newest therapeutics, such as natalizumab (anti-VLA-4), campath (anti-CD52), and fingolimod seem more promising, their eventual efficacy in the long run has still to be proven. Of course, any effective treatment is critical to prevent chronicity and progression of the disease, but there are no therapies to prevent the later stages of the disease.

In addition, the argument concerning the presence of autoantibodies and autoreactive T cells deserves scrutiny. Responses to myelin and neuronal proteins are also observed in healthy individuals and their presence in MS is not synonymous with disease. Also, if the hypothesis of a positive feedback loop with increasing damage as the disease progresses were correct, one would expect increasing titres of autoantibodies and determinant spreading if this phenomenon occurs at all; this is not the case.

The histology of the disease is also questionable. The scanty number of T cells in the lesions is hardly compatible with a direct damaging role for these cells. It is more than likely that damage occurs prior to this. The findings in the grey matter add more doubts to the autoimmune hypothesis, as demyelination seems to occur in the absence of inflammatory activity. Also, brain atrophy and neuronal loss progress relentlessly, in spite of anti-inflammatory treatments, suggesting that MS has important neurodegenerative aspects. This is as important as the inflammatory events involved in the initial stages, but probably not initiation of the disease. It is time to scrutinise the long-held dogma of MS as an autoimmune disease and examine in depth the potential neurodegenerative phenomena in MS.

The above can be taken as an encouragement to look at therapeutic options, other than immunosuppressive regimens. Studies on mitochondrial functions and abnormalities in MS are coming to the fore and suggest that there might be something in antioxidant therapies, even though such approaches in other neurodegenerative diseases have not met with great success yet. Though it is not clear whether oxidative stress is a cause or consequence of the disease, it is conceivable that preventing oxidative stress might ameliorate the disease course by abrogating the amplification of the damage that secondary oxidative stress brings.

In a disease that is characterised by the disappearance of myelinating cells, replenishing oligodendrocytes might also be considered an option and efforts are being made to develop stem cell therapies. The problems with an approach like this are huge and will not only involve getting enough stem cells to repair the damage, getting the stem cells to the right place, and getting them to differentiate at the right time and place, but will probably also require manipulating the local microenvironment, as this may be hostile to the newly arriving stem cells.

Another, but even more distant, option is to harness the brain's defence mechanisms against disease progression. The pre-active lesions described above occur with such frequency at any stage of the disease that it is almost unthinkable that all pre-active lesions will progress to active lesions. If that were the case one simply would have no normal white matter left in a few months to years. So, somehow the brain manages to redress a portion of pre-active lesions. If we could find out how the brain achieves this we could think of manipulating this mechanism to stop formation of new lesions altogether. Unfortunately we still have no idea what really triggers the occurrence of pre-active lesions, but this does seem a worthwhile avenue to explore.

Clearly, most of this is for the future. But it is good to realise that old dogmas need to be reassessed, and there may be more to MS than autoimmunity.

References

1. Dean, G. and Elian, M. (1997). Age at immigration to England of Asian and Caribbean immigrants and the risk of developing multiple sclerosis. *J. Neurol. Neurosurg. Psychiatry* **63**, 565–568.

2. Lucchinetti, C.F., Brück, W., Rodriguez, M., and Lassmann, H. (1996). Distinct patterns of multiple sclerosis pathology indicates heterogeneity on pathogenesis. *Brain Pathol.* **6**, 259–274.

3. Jankosky, C., Deussing, E., Gibson, R.L., and Haverkos, H.W. (2012). Viruses and vitamin D in the etiology of type 1 diabetes mellitus and multiple sclerosis. *Virus Res.*, in press.

4. Atkins, G.J., McQuaid, S., Morris-Downes, M.M., *et al.* (2000). Transient virus infection and multiple sclerosis. *Rev. Med. Virol.* **10**, 291–303.

5. Munger, K.L. and Ascherio, A. (2011). Prevention and treatment of MS: studying the effects of vitamin D. *Mult. Scler. J.* **17**, 1405–1411.

6. Sawcer, S., Hellenthal, G., Pirinen, M., Spencer, C.C.A., Donnelly, P., and Compston, A. (2011). Genetic risk and a primary role for cell-mediated immune mechanisms in multiple sclerosis. *Nature* **476**, 214–219.

7. Krakowski M. and Owens T. (1996). Interferon-gamma confers resistance to experimental allergic encephalomyelitis. *Eur. J. Immunol.* **26**, 1641–1646.

8. Tran, E.H., Prince, E.N., and Owens, T. (2000). IFN-gamma shapes immune invasion of the central nervous system via regulation of chemokines. *J. Immunol.* **164**, 2759–2768.

9. Cua, D.J., Sherlock, J., Chen, Y., *et al.* (2003). Interleukin-23 rather than interleukin-12 is the critical cytokine for autoimmune inflammation of the brain. *Nature* **421**, 744–748.

10. Komiyama, Y., Nakae, S., Matsuki, T., *et al.* (2006). IL-17 plays an important role in the development of experimental autoimmune encephalomyelitis. *J. Immunol.* **177**, 566–573.

11. Langrish, C.L., Chen, Y., Blumenschein, W.M., *et al.* (2005). IL-23 drives a pathogenic T cell population that induces autoimmune inflammation. *J. Exp. Med.* **201**, 233–240.

12. Matusevicius, D., Kivisakk, P., He, B., *et al.* (1999). Interleukin-17 mRNA expression in blood and CSF mononuclear cells is augmented in multiple sclerosis. *Mult. Scler.* **5**, 101–104.

13. Vaknin-Dembinsky, A., Balashov, K., and Weiner, H.L. (2006). IL-23 is increased in dendritic cells in multiple sclerosis and

down-regulation of IL-23 by antisense oligos increases dendritic cell IL-10 production. *J. Immunol.* **176**, 7768–7774.

14. Sutton, C., Brereton, C., Keogh, B., Mills, K.H., and Lavelle, E.C. (2006). A crucial role for interleukin (IL)-1 in the induction of IL-17-producing T cells that mediate autoimmune encephalomyelitis. *J. Exp. Med.* **203**, 1685–1691.

15. Brereton, C.F., Sutton, C.E., Lalor, S.J., Lavelle, E.C., and Mills, K.H. (2009). Inhibition of ERK MAPK suppresses IL-23- and IL-1-driven IL-17 production and attenuates autoimmune disease. *J. Immunol.* **183**, 1715–1723.

16. Kapsenberg, M.L. (2009). Gammadelta T cell receptors without a job. *Immunity* **31**, 181–183.

17. Sutton, C.E., Lalor, S.J., Sweeney, C.M., Brereton, C.F., Lavelle, E.C., and Mills, K.H. (2009). Interleukin-1 and IL-23 induce innate IL-17 production from gammadelta T cells, amplifying Th17 responses and autoimmunity. *Immunity* **31**, 331–341.

18. Lalor, S.J., Dungan, L., Sutton, C.E., Basdeo, S.A., Fletcher, J.M., and Mills, K.H.G. (2011). Caspase-1 processed cytokines IL-1β and IL-18 promote IL-17-production by γδ and CD4 T cells that mediate autoimmunity. *J. Immunol.* **186**, 5738–5748.

19. Veldhoen, M., Hocking, R.J., Flavell, R.A., and Stockinger, B. (2006). Signals mediated by transforming growth factor-beta initiate autoimmune encephalomyelitis, but chronic inflammation is needed to sustain disease. *Nat. Immunol.* **7**, 1151–1156.

20. Korn, T., Bettelli, E., Gao, W., *et al.* (2007). IL-21 initiates an alternative pathway to induce proinflammatory T(H)17 cells. *Nature* **448**, 484–487.

21. Kurzeja, M., Rudnicka, L., and Olszewska, M. (2011). New interleukin-23 pathway inhibitors in dermatology: ustekinumab, briakinumab, and secukinumab. *Am. J. Clin. Dermatol.* **12**, 113–125.

22. Chen, Y., Langrish, C.L., McKenzie, B., *et al.* (2006). Anti-IL-23 therapy inhibits multiple inflammatory pathways and ameliorates autoimmune encephalomyelitis. *J. Clin. Invest.* **116**, 1317–1326.

23. Segal, B.M., Constantinescu, C.S., Raychaudhuri, A., Kim, L., Fidelus-Gort, R., and Kasper, L.H. (2008). Repeated subcutaneous injections of IL12/23 p40 neutralising antibody, ustekinumab, in patients with relapsing-remitting multiple sclerosis: a phase II, double-blind, placebo-controlled, randomised, dose-ranging study. *Lancet Neurol.* **7**, 796–804.

24. Polman, C.H., O'Connor, P.W., Havrdova, E., *et al.* (2006). A randomized, placebo-controlled trial of natalizumab for relapsing multiple sclerosis. *N. Engl. J. Med.* **354**, 899–910.

25. Langer-Gould, A., Atlas, S.W., Green, A.J., Bollen, A.W., and Pelletier, D. (2005). Progressive multifocal leukoencephalopathy in a patient treated with natalizumab. *N. Engl. J. Med.* **353**, 375–381.

26. Coles, A.J., Compston, D.A., Selmaj, K.W., *et al.* (2008). Alemtuzumab vs. interferon beta-1a in early multiple sclerosis. *N. Engl. J. Med.* **359**, 1786–1801.

27. Keane, J., Gershon, S., Wise, R.P., *et al.* (2001). Tuberculosis associated with infliximab, a tumor necrosis factor alpha-neutralizing agent. *N. Engl. J. Med.* **345**, 1098–1104.

28. Sweeney, C.M., Lonergan, R., Basdeo, S.A., *et al.* (2011). IL-27 mediates the response to IFN-beta therapy in multiple sclerosis patients by inhibiting Th17 cells. *Brain Behav. Immun.* **25**, 1170–1181.

29. Stephens, L.A., Malpass, K.H., and Anderton, S.M. (2009). Curing CNS autoimmune disease with myelin-reactive Foxp3+ Treg. *Eur. J. Immunol.* **39**, 1108–1117.

Index

Printed in the United States
By Bookmasters